RATIONING: CONSTRUCTED R
PROFESSIONAL PRACTICES

T0220987

Sociology of Health and Illness Monograph Series

Edited by Jonathan Gabe
Department of Social and Political Science
Royal Holloway
Egham
Surrey
TW20 0EX
UK

Current titles:

- **Rethinking the Sociology of Mental Health (2000)**,
  edited by *Joan Busfield*
- **Sociological Perspectives on the New Genetics (1999)**
  edited by *Peter Conrad and Jonathan Gabe*
- **The Sociology of Health Inequalities (1998)**,
  edited by *Mel Bartley, David Blane and George Davey Smith*
- **The Sociology of Medical Science (1997)**,
  edited by *Mary Ann Elston*
- **Health and the Sociology of Emotion (1996)**,
  edited by *Veronica James and Jonathan Gabe*
- **Medicine, Health and Risk (1995)**,
  edited by *Jonathan Gabe*

Forthcoming titles:

Partners in Health, Partners in Crime
Explorations of the relationship between criminology and sociology of health and health care
Edited by Stefan Timmermans and Jonathan Gabe

Health and the Media
Edited by Clive Seale

Rationing
Constructed Realities and Professional Practices

Edited by

David Hughes & Donald Light

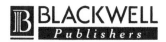

Copyright © Blackwell Publishers 2002

First published as volume 23, issue 5 of *Sociology of Health and Illness*, 2001

Blackwell Publishers Ltd
108 Cowley Road
Oxford OX4 1JF
UK

Blackwell Publishers Inc
350 Main Street
Malden, Massachusetts 02148
USA

British Library Cataloguing in Publication Data
A CIP catalogue record for this book is available from the British Library.

Library of Congress Cataloging in Publication Data has been applied for

ISBN: 0-631-22857-9-8

Contents

Notes on Contributors

Gary Albrecht is Professor of Public Health and of Disability and Human Development at the University of Illinois at Chicago. His most recent books are: *The Handbook of Social Studies in Health and Medicine* edited with Ray Fitzpatrick and Susan Scrimshaw (London: Sage, 2000) *and The Handbook of Disability Studies* edited with Katherine Seelman and Michael Bury (Thousand Oaks, CA: Sage 2001).

Hugh Armstrong is a Professor of Social Work and Political Economy at Carleton University. With Pat Armstrong, he has written widely on women and work and on health care. Their books *include The Double Ghetto: Canadian Women and Their Segregated Work* (Third Edition, 1994); *Wasting Away* (1996); and *Universal Health Care* (1998). With David Coburn, they *edited Unhealthy Times: Political Economy Perspectives on Health and Care in Canada* (2001).

Pat Armstrong is a Professor of Sociology at York University, Canada, and holds a CHSRF/CIHR chair in health services research. She has co-authored numerous books on health care including *Heal Thyself: Managing Health Care Reform*; *Wasting Away: The Undermining of Canadian Health Care*; *Universal Health Care: What the United States Can Learn From Canada*; *Vital Signs: Nursing in Transition*; and *Take Care: Warning Signals for Canada's Health System*.

Ivy Bourgeault is an Assistant Professor in Sociology and Health Sciences at the University of Western Ontario in London, Ontario, Canada. She holds a CIHR New Investigator Award for a five-year study of the impact of gender and geography on the rationalisation of the health care division of labour in Canada and the United States. Ivy has published extensively on midwifery and maternity care, the relations between health professions and the state, alternative medicine and patient consumerism.

Elizabeth Boyd is a Joint Postdoctoral Fellow at the Institute for Health Policy Studies at the University of California, San Francisco and the Veterans Administration Health Services Research and Development Program, Menlo Park, California. Her research interests include the patient-provider relation-hip, evidence-based medicine, and the ethics of clinical research.

Jacqueline Choiniere is the Director of Policy, Practice and Research of the Registered Nurses Association of Ontario. She is pursuing her PhD in

viii   Notes on Contributors

Sociology at York University and has been involved in several book projects with the Armstrongs and others including *Vital Signs: Nursing in Transition*; *Take Care: Warning Signals for the Canadian Health Care System*; *Medical Alert: New Work Organizations in Health Care*, and *Heal Thyself*.

Lesley Griffiths is a Senior Lecturer in Health Policy and Research at the University of Wales, Swansea. She has carried out a number of funded research projects for various bodies including the ESRC, Welsh Office of Research and Development and the Nuffield Trust. Her main interests lie in the areas of health communication, policy implementation and the use of ethnographic methods.

John Heritage is Professor of Sociology at UCLA. He is the author of *Garfinkel and Ethnomethodology*, and *The News Interview: Journalists and Public Figures On the Air* (with Steven Clayman), and the editor of *Structures of Social Action* (with Max Atkinson), *Talk at Work* (with Paul Drew), and *Practicing Medicine* (with Douglas Maynard). He is currently working on a range of topics in doctor-patient interaction, and on presidential press conferences (with Steven Clayman).

David Hughes is a Professor in the School of Health Science at the University of Wales Swansea and Dean of the Faculty of Education and Health Studies. His current research interests include the reformed NHS, health care rationing and the changing division of health labour. He has written on a range of topics in the fields of medical sociology, socio-legal studies and health policy.

Paul Joyce, Ph.D. is a Research Fellow at the University of Salford. His research interests include the management of expertise within organisational systems, in particular health care systems, and the use of virtual reality models in urban regeneration schemes. Currently, he is working on a project looking at the use of virtual learning environments to support under-graduate and postgraduate studies.

Lawrence C. Kleinman is a paediatrician and health services researcher who is a national expert on measuring and improving the quality of health care. An alumnus of Rutgers College, Bowman Gray School of Medicine, and UCLA School of Public Health, Dr. Kleinman was a Robert Wood Johnson Clinical Scholar at UCLA. He is a recipient of the Association for Health Services Research Article of the Year Award for his survey of the health of homeless adults in Los Angeles, and has published widely on topics ranging from the appropriateness of medical care to physician advocacy, and the history of public health.

Irvine Lapsley is Professor of Accounting and Director of the Institute of Public Sector Accounting Research at the University of Edinburgh. He is editor of *Financial Accountability & Management*, a research journal which specialises in public sector accounting issues. He has undertaken research on a variety of aspects of health care, including management structures, accounting controls and performance measurement and has published widely on these issues.

Joel Lexchin holds Associate Professorships in the Department of Family and Community Medicine at the University of Toronto and the School of Health Policy and Management at York University, Canada, and is an emergency physician at the University Health Network. He has written over 40 articles on pharmaceutical policy and prescribing, as well as two books on the pharmaceutical industry. He is one of three authors of *Drugs of Choice: A Formulary for General Practice*.

Donald W. Light is the Professor of comparative health care systems at the University of Medicine and Dentistry of New Jersey and a fellow at the Center for Bioethics at the University of Pennsylvania. Trained as a sociologist at the University of Chicago and Brandeis, he is a Faculty Associate in the Department of Sociology at Princeton University. Professor Light has written about distributive justice in the BMJ and is co-author of *Benchmarks of Fairness for Health Care Reform* (Oxford 1996).

Kath Melia, a nurse/sociologist, is Professor of Nursing Studies at the University of Edinburgh. She has published in the areas of sociology of health care professions and nursing ethics. She has recently undertaken research concerning ethics in intensive care, which raised questions about teamwork and the re-drawing of professional boundaries.

Eric Mykhalovskiy is a Lecturer and Postdoctoral Fellow in the Department of Public Health Sciences, Faculty of Medicine, University of Toronto. His publications and research address such questions as the social presence of evidentiary knowledge in contemporary health care reform, inter-textuality and health care reform, the critique of health services research, and the social organisation of health work done by people living with HIV/AIDS.

Elizabeth Suzanne Peters is a doctoral candidate in Sociology at York University, Canada, and an Associate Fellow of Winters College, York University, Canada. Her dissertation research is focused on theorising the nexus of governmentality, time and space in health care regimes. A health care professional, herself, Suzanne has a decade of experience working with populations with multiple health needs during the de-institutionalisation period in the Ontario health care regime.

Lindsay Prior is Reader in Sociology at Cardiff University, and Research Director of a joint UWCM/ Cardiff University programme on health and risk. His most recent journal papers have been on chronic fatigue syndrome, and lay accounts of health among Cantonese speakers in England. He has previously published books on the social organisation of death and on the social organisation of mental illness. His next book (to be published 2002) is concerned with the use of documents in social research.

Carine Vassy is Senior Lecturer in Sociology at the University of Paris 13, France. She leads the "Politics and Health" research group of the "Centre de Recherche pour les Enjeux de Santé Publique" (Center of Research for Public Health). Her current research interests are medical sociology, organisations and genetics.

Jerry White is Graduate Sociology Chair at the University of Western Ontario in London, Ontario, Canada. Jerry has authored a series of health-care books including collaborative works such as *Take Care*, *Medical Alert* and *Heal Thyself* and sole authorships like *Hospital Strike*. His research has been published internationally and covers diverse issues from nursing to Aboriginal population outcomes.

1

Introduction
A sociological perspective on rationing: power, rhetoric and situated practices

Donald W. Light and David Hughes

The analytic power of sociology stems from examining closely the deep structures and power relations that underlie the rhetorics and practices of individuals, groups and organisations, by assuming a radical disengagement from them. Such is the analytic promise of sociological research into rationing, where unexamined rhetoric prevails and detailed empirical studies are thin on the ground. Intellectuals and policy makers, as well as those who pay the bills – be they governmental bodies, employers, insurers, or individuals – need the unclouded gaze of the sociological eye more than ever, as the rhetorics of rationing swirl around them. For rationing has become a predominant issue in the economic, moral and political discourses on health care. Yet as Conrad and Brown (1993:3) observed, 'rationing has received little sociological attention'.

The sociological perspective has much to offer. At a time when scholarly thinking about rationing is dominated by the discipline of economics, sociology can help us to understand how economic transactions are embedded in social relations (Granovetter, 1985), which place limits on calculative rationality. Rationing provides a valuable array of social practices for exploring power relations in health care systems, particularly the linkage between resource allocation, rhetoric and the interests of different parties. Sociological studies can also complement and extend philosophical and ethical work on rationing by providing empirical case material grounded in the practical circumstances of real-world decision making, and investigating whether the ethical issues recognised by actors in the health care system correspond with those described in the scholarly literature. Our aim as editors was to put together a volume that would start to address some of these issues, and we think that a decade from now one will find that an important body of research has been achieved.

The fallacy of inevitable rationing

As rationing has gained prominence in intellectual and policy circles, one increasingly hears that it has always been there, like Monsieur Jourdain in Moliere's *Le Bourgeois Gentilhomme*, who learns that he has been speaking prose all his life. For example, a widely-read article on the subject begins by stating that: 'Medical care has always been rationed by the supply available, by its distribution, and by the public's ability to pay' (Mechanic 1995: 1655). But what, exactly, does this mean? Was it rationed even in the decades when numerous studies documented in the United States surpluses of doctors and hospital beds, as well as large portions of excessive and unnecessary tests, prescriptions, operations, hospital admissions and bed days? (We will get to the uninsured later.) Still more broadly, a leading moral philosopher writes, 'Whenever we design institutions that distribute these goods, and whenever we operate those institutions, we are involved in rationing' (Daniels 1994: 27). If rationing always takes place, does that mean one cannot imagine a state in which medical care is not rationed?

Our selection of this topic for the monograph reflects our belief that rationing is a crucial issue in contemporary health care systems, and at the present time a pervasive process. However, we argue that a proper sociological analysis cannot assume that rationing arises straightforwardly as a necessary part of resource allocation per se. Arguably, rationing is not simply a product of an imbalance between supply and demand, but is also shaped by a layering of cultural beliefs and social organisation. David Hunter (1997: 20) hints at what we have in mind when he writes: 'So, given how politicians and public conceive of the issue, rationing, priority-setting, making choices, or whatever term is preferred, is inevitable at least to *some* degree...' Arguably, 'conceptions' are crucial. Rationing is not an invariant economic fact (although there are circumstances where it may be inescapable), but rather a central component of contemporary political and social discourses on the allocation of health care resources.

We argue that the concept of rationing is to a large extent a rhetorical construction: it formulates a particular linkage between allocative decisions and resources which can work to support certain interests against others. It is a way of framing reality that came to prominence in Western countries in the late 20th century, and which constructs the nature of resource allocation processes differently from the discourses of the past (see: Joyce, in this volume). A sociological research agenda must incorporate many previously neglected questions: what different stakeholders mean by 'rationing', what criteria they invoke when they say it is happening, what agenda they have in advancing their arguments, and what practitioners actually do and how they understand the reality they construct. We will first examine some of the prominent rhetorics, and then show how deeply 'rationing' is a socially constructed reality, before introducing the collection of original investigations that make up this volume.

Parsing the rhetorics of rationing

Behind the increasing prevalence of statements that 'rationing is inevitable' lies the world view of economic theory and the degree to which it is being taken up by political scientists, moral philosophers, policy-makers and politicians without sufficient examination. Economics is based on the assumption of scarcity: there is never enough of anything and therefore rationing is ubiquitous. Thus many economists equate rationing with choice, and assume that scarcity always exists and that priority-setting is an inherent part of rational choice (Begg *et al.* 1987). This too is a model-driven rhetoric, a mental construct that needs empirical examination and appears to be highly contestable, even within its own terms of reference.

Consider the basic model of modern microeconomics, taught around the world. That model assumes that all resources and services are scarce. Further, it asserts a 'principle of non-satiation', stating that people are never satisfied (Katz and Rosen 1991: Chapter 1). This guarantees scarcity, even of things that are abundant. Economic behaviour therefore focuses on how to deal with scarcity. The standard model assumes that people deal with scarcity by having preferences and by trying to maximise their preferences in rank order of priority (1991: Chapter 2). That is, rational choice is complete (one's preferences are clearly ranked and complete) and transitive (one prefers in rank order). Within the constructed world of the micro-economic model of reality, this leads to defining which combinations of trade-offs are equivalent so that one can plot an 'indifference curve' of points at which a person is indifferent about one combination or another. In short, rationing is inherent in all choices. If you choose to see a friend, whether you think about it or not (a sign of irrationality), you are choosing it over other things you would like to do and over seeing other friends in the same time-slot. Thus, maximising one's preferences, given their rankings and ratios, means maximising one's indifference curve until one reaches 'equilibrium', which is defined as reaching one's highest indifference curve within one's financial constraints or time constraints. Otherwise, one is wasting resources (time, money) and is acting irrationally.

So far, this model cannot predict or rank because no values have been assigned. This shortcoming is overcome by assigning 'utilities' to one's preferences. This allows one to calculate 'opportunity costs' which are the value of all the alternatives one might have chosen. It also allows one to write all the basic equations of microeconomics, their constants and slopes, so as to measure and predict all the choice/rationing tradeoffs inherent in the model.

There are intuitive and experiential reasons to question this model that underlies much modern economic policy analysis. Let us consider pure choice with no rationing consequences for others, choices with indirect consequences, and choices with direct consequences. If you go to a restaurant and choose the grilled bass, is this rationing? Clearly yes, says the dismal science. You have just foregone other entrées. Indeed we often weigh the choices offered by a menu and are very aware of what we have not chosen. What does the concept mean in these circumstances?

Now suppose you are at a family barbeque and you choose the pork chop, not the chicken or the burger, because you prefer it. The dismal science would point out that in choosing the chop, no one else can have it, a decision that has direct rationing consequences for others. Or does it? Suppose the other two did not want the pork chop in the first place?

'Would you like an aisle or window seat?' the airline reservationist asks. You like a window, but you don't like to climb over others to stretch or go to the toilet; so you choose an aisle seat. So far, this is like choosing the grilled bass, but suppose aisle seats are popular? Then your choice has indirect rationing consequences for others. Sociologically, how shall we understand such situations? Usually, they are more complex. For example, a number of patients on surgical waiting lists report that they pay privately for a consultation and then the consultant jumps them up and operates on them the next week. This is the low-cost way to get quick elective surgery, and of course it pushes everyone else back. Is this "rationing" and if so in what sense, with what organisational dynamics?

The assumption of non-satiation needs examination. There is a five-day holiday coming up; shall we fly to a sun-dappled beach or go visit grandma who lives across the country? Shall the government allocate more for education, or more for health care? Does it matter that we have been able both to visit grandma and get away to a beach in the past several months? Does it matter how big the budget is for education and for health care? The implication is that calling these 'rationing' is based on thinking, 'But the budget could always be bigger' or 'You can't do everything all at once'. Priority setting need not be considered rationing, unless so declared.

Is enough never enough, by definition, even when people seemed quite satisfied? For example, a number of countries seem to have provided virtually all the health care that patients want or need in a timely manner for decades (Light 1997b). There is a bottom to the so-called bottomless pit of demand for health care, because people do have other things they like to do with their lives besides go to doctors and enter hospitals. In fact, many people shun them. To say that rationing 'always exists' or is 'inevitable', then, must be true by definition. As stated in a *British Medical Journal* round-up on rationing, 'Scarcity leads to a need to choose what to purchase and what not to purchase (that is, rationing)' (Donaldson 1996). 'I'll take the pork chop'. Thus 'rationing is inevitable' could be replaced with 'choice is inevitable' without missing a logical beat. Yet what a difference! The fallacy of defining a term as referring to nearly everything and being pervasive and inevitable is that it tells us nothing. The world is ready, in short, for a more differentiated, grounded and empirical account of what 'rationing' means and how it is carried out.

A sociological approach would be radically empirical about the claims of the microeconomic model. What preferences do people, or organisations or governments have, and how do they employ them in making choices with economic consequences? To what extent do they weigh and rank their preferences, or jump around, or use different frames in intermingled ways? To what extent do they estimate, or even think about, the "opportunity costs" of what they have chosen not to do as they choose what to do? (Planners may point out that paying for a new costly drug that helps two per cent of patients could be used for a prevention programme in heart disease that would benefit 22 per cent, but are budgetary discussions carried on this way?) To the extent that people do not weigh and rank within a consistent frame, the concept of rationing has no logical basis and invocations of 'rationing' need to be understood in other ways.

Continua and rationing decisions

One possible solution to this definitional problem is to reframe rationing as a form of collective planning that suppresses individual choice. We might say that rationing happens when people are denied scarce resources, which they would have chosen if given the opportunity, and which would have been of benefit to them. Many scholars maintain that health care rationing only occurs when a person is denied a treatment or service that s/he needed and/or which would have been of benefit. How far does this rescue the argument about the economic inevitability of rationing?

The immediate problem that one encounters is that need or benefit must be measured on multiple dimensions, which generally do not share a common pattern. For example, Norman Daniels (1994), one of the most prominent moral philosophers of justice and rationing, argues that justifiable health care is limited to services that patients need and that are effective. In theory, this eliminates large volumes of demand, the growing number of drugs and operations that enhance normal capacities, and scores of ineffective tests or procedures. Yet each key term is surrounded by a continuum of ambiguity.

The need-demand continuum
The demand for most needed tests, drugs or procedures can be characterised as a triangle in which need fills the upper peak, demand fills the broad base and both become increasingly intermiingled as one moves towards the middle. However, the picture is not static. The concept, or at least practice, of professionally-certified need shifts as more services become available. No natural cut-off point is evident between rationing and non-rationing. One cannot identify a change in the pattern of need that allows one to draw a line where treatment should cease to be provided. Further, any plausible cut-off point will change as volume increases and expectations change. A good example would be the 'need' for hip or knee replacements. Even if clinical

criteria for need are developed, it is the sociological dynamics of this process, the social construction of eligibility criteria and local practices that will shape real allocative decisions.

The effective-ineffective continuum

Effectiveness, however defined, is relative and a continuous variable with no clear cut-off. Different parties may define 'rationing' in different ways amongst themselves, and between different modes of production or service. Adverse and side effects add further complexity to determining what is 'effective'. There is no point at which 'rationing' begins, and therefore, any claim of rationing is a socially or politically constructed reality. Most continua of effectiveness or cost-effectiveness are unlikely to be linear. The question remains, where does 'rationing' begin? and thus what medical care is 'necessary'?

Nor is this question answered by recent attempts to make rationing 'rational' by recasting it as a set of systematic techniques to guide allocative decisions. Two tools, which have been subjected to considerable study and refinement and aim to allocate resources so that the greatest benefit is enjoyed by the greatest number of people, are quality adjusted life years and its cousin, disability adjusted life years. QALYs and DALYs, however, pose a number of problems. For example, they discriminate against people with chronic conditions who are unlikely to get better or are even getting worse (Alzheimer's disease comes to mind), and they presume to compare apples, oranges and pears on the grounds that they are all fruit. Or, to put it more formally, it is not 'feasible to collapse the multifaceted phenomena of life and its quality on to a single valid scale' (Hunter 1997: 72). Any attempt to quantify the quality of people's lives will be biased in its measures and sample. There are a number of practical and technical problems as well (Hunter 1997: 70–73). The point at which taking away more or fewer QALYs from an individual or population constitutes rationing cannot be resolved by a technical formula. Does rationing begin when the first QALY is taken away from a population? Most of the time health decision makers do not even know if it is happening.

Much more significant in practice are the large-scale efforts to ground clinical practices in scientific medicine – the movement known as evidence-based medicine (EBM). Enthusiasts believe that EBM will minimise rationing, because all ineffective tests, drugs and procedures will be stopped and the money saved will pay for effective interventions (for example, Roberts *et al.* 1996). This theory sounds fine, though even at its best EBM will produce evidence of marginal gains, trade-offs between benefits and complications or harms, and evidentiary ambiguity. The problem of how benefits are measured, like measuring improved quality of life, arises again, as does the problem of transposing different kinds of benefits into one scale. How, for example, does one weigh reduced risk of death against increased chances of impotence in the treatment of cancer, and how does one scale what these trade-offs mean for different men? Further, women favour reduced risk of death over less sex, while male partners favour sexual activities more heavily. Such problems point to internal forms of rationing embedded in methods used, samples drawn, and scales constructed – all by a technological élite that is usually invisible and not accountable to the patients affected. If one surmounts these difficulties, one comes again to a spate of practical problems of implementing evidence-based medicine, starting with the low priority that doctors and even purchasers give to such evidence, and ending with the complexities of applying epidemiological evidence to individual cases (Tanenbaum 1994, Frankford 1994, Hunter 1997). In terms of rationing, EBM poses the same problems as those posed by "effectiveness". In the absence of natural cut-off points in much of the data on effectiveness and costs, it is unclear conceptually where rationing begins to occur or, if rationing is framed as a technical exercise, where different decision tools indicate that treatments should cease to be provided.

Does rationing happen in voluntary markets?

One anomaly in economic theories of scarcity occurs when rationing is claimed to be inevitable, yet price competition is not considered to be 'rationing'; for 'rationing' is used to refer to non-price ways of allocating scarce resources. Such decisions may be made by politicians or clinicians at either the micro or macro level (through writing national protocols), but their nature is economic. Further, such conscious and planned forms of allocation, through QALYs or clinical protocols, are presumed to be just and fair. When forms of rationing are advocated in favour of 'just letting things happen' or leaving doctors to make their autonomous decisions, it is usually provoked by evidence of mischief or untrustworthy behaviour. To put this in the terms of David Hume and his modern interpreter, Julian LeGrand (1997), rationing aims to eliminate knavish behaviours towards pawns and supplant them with knightly schemes. Indeed, rationing presumes paternalism and trust in the knights, while markets presume people are knaves and aim to curb their clever knaveries by pitting them against each other so that self-seeking behaviours work for the common good.

Especially in the United States, many regard the notion of 'rationing by price' as a contradiction in terms. If allocations occur through prices and markets, that is regarded as 'natural'. Somehow, the choice-is-rationing argument gets dropped, so that allocating scarce resources by price is acceptable, while planned mechanisms which restrict access to care are not, and rationing per se is an unnatural, contrived way of allocating scarce resources.

This argument is central to whether health-care rationing can be said to exist at all in the United States or other systems that lack a mechanism for providing universal access to health care. Some claim that it does, as when

Conrad and Brown (1993:11) write: '... one of the most disturbing examples of allocative rationing is the existence of roughly 37 million people without any health insurance'. We sympathise, and the number of uninsured, net of new people insured, has been rising by about 100,000 a month, every year since that time. But our sympathy rests on the premise that health insurance should be universal, not sold in a voluntary market that is ruled by the 'inverse coverage law' that has spawned a variety of ways to discriminate against those with health needs (Light 1992). Conrad and Brown probably share this assumption; but it is important to be clear that, given the logic of the voluntary health care market, this is not 'rationing'. In the United States, there is no general right to health care. Yet ambivalent feelings lead to Medicare, Medicaid and other public programmes, like food stamps and public housing, as specific interventions to deal with some forms of market failure in the mainstream private market.

Sociologists investigating denied services must take full proper account of the logic of the market and the way it frames reality. This is central to American-style managed care. Employers and governments have turned health care over to for-profit managed care corporations, to what Uwe Reinhardt (1996) calls in his colourful but insightful account 'bounty hunters'. Employers and governments, after years of failed efforts to get American physicians to help them restrain costs, hired corporate bounty hunters to 'shoot down' costs for rewards in the millions. Was this rationing? They 'shot down' very high fees and bed-day prices by forcing doctors and hospitals to take discounts. Both speak of 'rationing' but what does that mean, except 'less than we're used to having'? Some West Coast surgeons had their fees cut and saw their personal incomes plummet from $500,000 a year to $250,000. Was this rationing? American Medical Association data showed that, overall, physicians' incomes stopped rising and stayed flat. Hospitals claim that discounted payments 'ration' charity care, but even non-profit hospitals have done little charity care, and the percentage of gross revenues devoted to charity care has not dropped substantially. The bounty hunters also cut hospital admissions and shortened lengths of stay. Was this rationing or cutting into the fat of unnecessary hospitalisation?

HMOs (health maintenance organisations) and MCOs (managed care organisations) provide inferior care to patients who have chronic conditions, are elderly or are poor. They deny tests, hospital admissions, or operations, but is this 'rationing'? If we are seeking an authoritative definition of rationing, the answer is not clear. If the corporations use protocols based on effectiveness, even untested ones of their own choosing, or if the procedures are not covered in the particular health insurance policy of that particular patient, those involved may deny that rationing is occurring. The corporations have the same right as any corporation in a voluntary market to provide services according to the contractual terms specified. And yet for those who do not receive care, the results bear a close family resemblance to 'rationing' in other systems. Patients and their doctors often think the denials constitute rationing; but they do not seem to realise that this judgement presumes that health care is a right, when the US system assumes it is a commodity.

Getting inside the 'black box'

Given these definitional uncertainties how should policy makers, economists, researchers and moral philosophers proceed? Rationing takes place in several forms according to the most influential current literature: Diagnosis-related groups (DRGs), cost-sharing or user fees, capitation schemes, denial of services, fixed budgets, waiting lists and requirements for prior authorisation of treatments. We do not doubt that each of these might involve rationing, but they may not.

It depends on how actors conceive of 'rationing', and on actual practice and the details of what happens. Sociologically, what matters are the interactions, power relations, perspectives and agendas of the relevant parties. This is as relevant at the macro level of national political decisions, as it is at the meso level of US HMOs or British Primary Care Trusts, and the clinical micro-level. Thus the first research objective is to get inside the 'black box' of organisations at different levels of the health care system to gauge what is happening on the ground.

The need for an up-close look is all too apparent with some of the examples mentioned above. For example, in order to stop the relentless increases in procedures and charges, the US Congress created DRGs by taking the average practices and charges after 25 years of escalation and bundling them into a single payment per diagnostic-related group. As the largest payer, Congress was saying, 'You can live within the totals you have built up, and we will pay no more'. Was this 'rationing'? Hospitals reacted as if it were, by dramatically reducing lengths of stay, nursing staff and the like. Their profit margins soared as they complained about this draconian form of 'rationing' by Congress.

User fees clearly reduce front-end use of services that patients control. Studies show they reduce in about equal proportions both unnecessary and needed services. They are a crude instrument that discriminates by class, but at what point might one say they are 'rationing'? How many of the needed services are effective?

Capitation schemes, like DRGs writ large, are based on historic patterns of utilisation and charges driven up during the decades of fee for service, and the questions are the same. If providers limit access or treatments within capitation contracts, especially US-sized ones, one needs to look more to the providers and their motives than capitation schemes per se.

Across the Atlantic, waiting lists seem to some like an inherent form of rationing, because everyone on them has been seen by a qualified clinician and deemed to need the service or treatment. But what is being rationed, especially if everyone is ultimately treated? The most likely candidates are waiting itself, perhaps suffering, anxiety, the impaired ability to carry out a full life, and the reduced risk of increased morbidity or mortality that early treatment might bring.

Other 'grey areas' in the UK context include prior authorisation of extra contractual referrals (ECRs) in the NHS internal market, and restrictions on the prescribing of 'life-style drugs such as Viagra (Redwood 2000). In the 'Child B' case, a health authority that had refused to fund a second bone-marrow transplant as an ECR argued that it did so because expert medical opinion suggested that the chance of a successful outcome was minimal. Subsequently, 'Child B' obtained the desired treatment by other means but lived for only a short time. Yet many thought cost had been a factor in the decision and accusations of rationing persisted. Viagra, and more recently the anti-obesity drug Orlistat, were regarded by many British health authorities as medically unnecessary drugs that would not normally be purchased from core budgets. However, some observers argue that these drugs are prescribed for health-damaging conditions, and that a blanket ban which ignores individual patients' circumstances constitutes rationing. The National Institute of Clinical Excellence, the institution set up by the UK Government in 1999 to provide national guidelines on the clinical effectiveness of particular interventions, issued guidance on Orlistat in March 2001, setting out a fairly narrow range of circumstances in which the drug should be prescribed, but has not so far considered Viagra. In all these cases the factors which shape decisions require close empirical examination. Although the presence or absence of rationing is likely to remain a contentious issue, we need to know more about how actors weigh the various factors and whether they perceive that a rationing process is at work.

One test of where rationing begins is to ask: 'under what conditions would you say there is no rationing?' Would this be the case if everyone were seen the same day they were referred, or the same week, or month?' This question can be applied to all the assertions about rationing. At the macro level, how big would the budget have to be before those who claim that the government or programme is rationing would agree that no more rationing is taking place? At the meso level, how many hospitals, how close together, would there have to be before a given stakeholder, or policy analyst, would say that geographical rationing is not taking place? Less than a 60-minute bus ride? Less than 30 minutes? Less than 15? How short would waiting times have to be? Of course, different observers will answer these questions in different ways. They will make a case for drawing the line in one place rather than another, or perhaps talk of grey areas where they acknowledge that it is hard to say. We are brought back once again to the micro-politics of rationing as a struggle over definitions, reflecting different situated interests and perspectives.

Power relations in rationing

Economic concepts of rationing as reasoned choice, or a set of techniques for the rational allocation of resources, tend to obscure the underlying power relationships involved. Whether allocation decisions are made by politicians, managers, doctors or intellectuals, the typical pattern is that a small group of élite actors ration services for others. It is true that decisions about priorities and trade-offs might be made in a more transparent and participatory way (Daniels *et al.* 1996), but in practice such initiatives rarely amount to anything more than short-term experiments. More apparent is an ongoing power struggle in which politicians, policy makers, managers, clinicians and analysts try to justify or challenge allocative decisions. The rhetorics of rationing can be used to support arguments for both less care and more care. Politicians and managers can use it to justify reduced services and budgets, especially for the most vulnerable, in order to advance their own agendas on other fronts. Other managers and clinicians may try to use the 'R' word to mobilise public opposition to service reductions or failure to provide new services. Allegations of rationing can be seen as a particularly powerful form of claims-making activity (Spector and Kitsuse 1977), which at the extreme may lead the public to recognise a new social problem. Thus the use of rationing as political rhetoric is another fit subject for incisive research.

Rationing rests on the belief that those in power have the best interests of their subjects in mind and that one can trust them to allocate scarce resources fairly. Such beliefs are actually empirical questions to be researched. Waiting lists, for example, rest on the public's trust that doctors choose whom to treat next in terms of clinical needs, suffering and life circumstances; but there is little evidence that this is the case. Thus the correlation between long waiting lists and large private practices among surgeons, together with a contract that provides strong incentives to build up one's private practice (perhaps by encouraging long waiters to 'go private'), indicate that power is not always paternalistic (Yates 1996, Light 2000a).

These conceptual points pertain directly to a favourite subject of debate, whether rationing should be implicit or explicit. This issue arises, as Mechanic (1993), Hunter (1997), and Griffiths and Hughes (1998) describe, because governments throughout the world have needed to hold down costs on public services and have turned to new modes of purchasing. In a brief history of the origins of managed care (Light 1997a), this is characterised as 'the buyers' revolt' because payers who had passively paid the rising medical bills for years started acting like active buyers. Whatever rationing took place before was implicit, and the argument is that purchasing requires one to be explicit about what services one wants, at what levels of quality and error rates, not unlike Ford purchasing differentials or door handles.

This movement has led, inter alia, to systematic efforts at both the local and national level to compare the outcomes of specified clinical procedures, define standards, collate scientific evidence on the effectiveness of procedures, tests and medicines, and develop guidelines about whether these should be purchased. Nevertheless, some of the best minds in the social sciences, like David Mechanic, Rudolf Klein and David Hunter, have issued warnings about explicit rationing and written in favour of implicit rationing. Many of their warnings are political; explicit rationing of health care will provoke the public and may tie health care policy into knots. They also emphasise the need to consider the highly variable circumstances and clinical conditions of patients who otherwise have the same disorder that would be subjected to the same protocol or explicit rule.

These critics make powerful points about the limitations of formal schemes of rationing. What their arguments can overlook, however, is that implicit rationing by doctors has been rife with evidence of large, unexplained variations, of unnecessary expenditures and of uneven quality because physicians put their autonomy and interests ahead of patients. That is, professional power and autonomy have too often not been exercised in trustworthy ways that manifest the application of medical science to the best interests of patients. Any arguments for the merits of implicit rationing must address these problems. While it is true that 'doctors' specialist knowledge remains irreplaceable, which itself places limits on managers' incursions into medical territory' (Hunter 1997: 56), specialists' knowledge can be – and is – subjected to clinical standards, guidelines and protocols developed by teams of specialists. It is the engineers at Ford who develop the 'specs' for purchasing differentials, not the managers. The key to a solution, we believe, lies in re-conceptualising professionalism around accountability rather than autonomy; so that the use of power in both explicit and implicit rationing are subject to transparent review. The theoretical point is that rationing of both kinds involves power, but accountability is more effective than trust to keep the best interests of patients in focus.

Researching the social construction of 'rationing'

Every day in every health care system, people are turned away, denied services, discharged quickly from hospital, made to pay at least part of the bill, and told that desired treatments are not covered. Budget directors and executives decide how much to spend, how much to allocate to one service or another, and how to pay for them. Lines are drawn in the distributional ambiguities of each of our theoretical continua. This is fertile ground for sociological studies to investigate what these actors do and what they think they are doing. How do they talk about resource allocation and conceptualise it? What rules do they apply? When do they fall silent? How can we deconstruct these discourses to understand them? What technologies are developed, by whom, with what kinds of biases built in? Organisationally, who is involved and at what levels? To what extent are the limited choices and resources at the clinical level determined by upstream choices that become the taken-for-granted context in which services are delayed or denied (Light 1997b)?

Another set of research questions is posed by philosophers thinking about the nature of rationing. For example, Daniels (1994) identifies three analytic features of rationing situations. Sometimes, goods or services come in chunks that cannot be divided and distributed, so that some people who ought to receive them do not. Second, benefits are denied to individuals who can make as plausible a claim on them based on principle as those who receive them. And third, principles of fair distribution do not allow one to choose among claimants. A research question for sociologists, who could contribute to moral deliberations, is to what degree do parties and organisations recognise these features, and if so, how do they deal with them? Daniels also poses problems of rationing which moral philosophers have to date been unable to solve. How much should we favour best outcomes in allocating resources and thus disfavour those unlikely to improve? Second, how much priority should be given to the neediest? Third, how shall we weigh modest benefits to many against significant benefits to a few? And to what extent should we rely on democratic processes to determine what kinds of rationing are fair? The research question again is to what extent do actors and institutions recognise these problems, and if so, how do they address them. How, for example, are concepts such as 'the neediest' defined in real-world situations? Moral philosophers raise questions and make distinctions not made in economics or any other discipline, and they can deepen the sociological research agenda.

This vast and seminal field needs sociological research to elucidate practices and principles. The studies reported in this volume start to address some, though not all, of the issues mapped out above. They consider the allocation of health care resources at both the macro and micro levels, using data from North America and Europe. Although the salience of rationing varies as one moves between levels and settings, it is rarely far beneath the surface. As Joyce shows, the rhetoric of rationing now features explicitly in the everyday discourses of British health care managers and their discussions with senior clinicians (see also: Griffiths and Hughes 1998; 2000). In the past, the term 'rationing' seems to have been rarely used by physicians themselves, even in the NHS, where it has been argued that doctors have traditionally presented what were essentially economic decisions as decisions taken on clinical grounds (Aaron and Schwartz 1984, Klein 1990), but this too may be changing.

Certainly, references to resources are beginning to feature explicitly in collegial interactions, as well as in the more reflexive context of the research interview. The clinical geneticists studied by Prior do not routinely talk of rationing in their everyday clinic work, but resources are a factor that must be considered when senior colleagues fix the risk thresholds that will trigger more intensive interventions, and in interviews these doctors state that a rationing process is at work. The French emergency department staff observed by Vassy speak of 're-directing' patients rather than denying treatment, but they are well aware that this is what may be involved and relax departmental rules to provide care for disadvantaged yet deserving patients who are not technically emergency cases. Across the Atlantic, the nurses interviewed by Bourgeault and associates again point to a clear link between resource constraints and limits on care. Policies on care pathways and early discharge that others may portray in terms of effectiveness and efficiency are seen by nurses as cost-cutting exercises that reduce the quality and quantity of the service. These are perceived as a threat to patient welfare and, one suspects, also as an imposed and unwelcomed change to the nature of nursing work.

Vassy suggests that contemporary studies of rationing can build on the conceptual foundations laid by an earlier generation of sociological studies concerned with client categorisation, screening and selection (see for example: Roth 1972, Sudnow 1965, Byrd 1981). In line with this older strand of organisational ethnography, Vassy investigates the informal rules of the emergency department in action, though with a more precise focus on the consequences of selection decisions (in terms of denied or delayed treatments). Micro-rationing takes place in a variety of focused interactions medical consultations, case conferences, ward rounds, telephone conversations between referring physicians and utilisation review staff for which sociologists now have well-developed techniques of analysis. Past studies show that clinicians move between multiple discourse frames as they try to make sense of patients and their work within a range of organisational and cultural contexts (Jeffrey 1979, Light 1980: Chapters 7–8, Frader and Bosk 1981). They fabricate discourses which interweave references to clinical criteria with locally-produced 'natural rhetorics' that point to factors such as deservingness and resource pressures (Griffiths and Hughes 1994, Hughes and Griffiths 1996).

In this volume Griffiths' research on British community mental health teams (CMHTs) illustrates how a preoccupation with resource constraints becomes entwined with concerns about disciplinary expertise and professional identity in the team context. Decisions about admission of patients onto caseloads are generally cast in terms of appropriateness rather than rationing, but staff make frequent references to the burden that inappropriate cases place on the CMHT and the need for better 'gatekeeping' by referring doctors. The question that Griffiths raises is whether patients get little or no care because they are 'inappropriate' cases, or if, in practice, the CMHT constructs certain cases as 'inappropriate' to exclude them and keep workload to a manageable level.

A second interactional study by Heritage, Boyd and Kleinman examines the delicate telephone negotiations between physician reviewers (employed by a utilisation review firm) and specialists who have recommended surgical insertion of tympanostomy tubes for child patients. It extends earlier work (Boyd 1998) which found that referring physicians could make denial less likely by emphasising their first-hand knowledge of the case and co-operating with the reviewer to recast the interaction as a bureaucratic formality in which they supplied necessary missing information. In this volume, Heritage and associates investigate the scope for bending UR firm rules by analysing talk concerning a significant subset of cases approved for surgery, even when the official criteria recommend against it. In outline they find that appeals to professional judgement by referring doctors can be successful in over-riding scientific, protocol-based decision making. In contrast to the strategies of deliberate 'gaming' described by some commentators (Morreim 1991, Freeman *et al.* 1999, Wynia *et al.* 2000), these doctors engage in a more subtle form of cultural resistance.

The theme of resistance surfaces in other chapters in the context of nurses (Bourgeault *et al.*), rank-and-file CMHT members (Griffiths) and patients (Albrecht, Prior). Arguably, Lapsley and Melia's account of 'soft rationing' in the ITU setting can also be seen in these terms. They are interested in how far clinicians can redefine the boundaries of the budgetary rules imposed upon them, and particularly how the impact of seemingly binding constraints can be attenuated by active clinical management and co-operative behaviour within social networks in the hospital and beyond. Soft rationing refers to a situation where general resource constraints still remain but are partially mitigated by a combination of flexible working practices and the willingness of clinicians to take risks by committing resources that may not be within budget. The argument parallels one made in earlier work on hard and soft contracting for social care services (Lapsley and Llewellyn 1997). Arguably this research points to a more general social process that occurs when the economics-based discourse of accounting and finance comes into contact with professional networks.

Lapsley and Melia, and Prior, make the point that economic conceptions of rationing set up an over-blunt dichotomy between treatment and denial, when what is at issue is more nuanced and uncertain. Many of the studies in this volume focus on a kind of grey area, where it is difficult to be sure of the consequences for patients of, say, a medium rather than high-risk genetics surveillance regime, or anxiety-management classes rather than full CMHT support, or 're-direction' from the ED to a community physician. In this zone of indeterminacy, managers, health professionals and patients may all recognise that denials and limitation of services are occurring, but perceive the results only dimly. Given the definitional uncertainties and the need to research this grey area, it makes sense to locate the sociology of rationing within a wider sociology of resource allocation. Thus some chapters in the present volume highlight the limits rather than the clear application of rationing processes.

Sociological studies of rationing, and resource allocation more generally, need to develop better methods to shed light on these issues. One strong feature of Heritage and associates' wider study is a combination of fine-grained process data with quantitative outcomes data. The addition of better outcomes data would undoubtedly have strengthened other inter-actional studies in this volume and is one direction for future development. Another way to illuminate the cumulative impact of rationing policies on individuals is to map patient biographies over time. Albrecht shows how, from the health consumer's perspective, the experience of rationing under managed care may not be just about the denial of one desired procedure (though this may indeed be critical), but a worrisome series of episodes in which, even when a treatment is given, required supporting services are not offered and problems arise over fees and reimbursement. One suspects that for groups such as socially-disadvantaged ED attenders or sufferers of 'non-serious' mental health problems, the experience of rationing centres not so much on a single denial decision but an ongoing mode of engagement with services and gatekeepers.

More broadly, several of the chapters link rationing to the theme of translations. As we argued earlier, the contemporary discourse on rationing can itself be seen as part of a wider translation in which thinking about health care systems is increasingly 're-coded' in terms of concepts from economic theory. Joyce identifies this specifically with neo-liberal ideas and associated formulae of governance, which re-interpret historic patterns of resource allocation as forms of implicit rationing and demand that this be supplanted by explicit rationing processes framed within the economics discourse. He points out that inter alia this involves a shift in the perception of individual and collective risk. Prior, as well, is clear that application of the rationing procedures and technologies devised to permit rational allocation requires specific translations of population data into personal risk, and of 'risk' into pathology. We might also point to the translation that occurs between the discourse of clinical medicine and the discourse of financial accounting. This is present in both US-style managed care and the NHS, but may take place closer to, or further from, the sites of clinical practice. Lapsley and Melia's work suggests that where models used for budgetary accounting purposes have little usefulness for prospective clinical decision making, doctors tend to push this translation back into the territory of the accountants. The authors describe how the ITU doctors agreed to a 'benchmarking exercise' to compare the performance of local ITU units, but wrote what might have been expected to be a financial audit document in clinical language, even relegating financial information to an appendix. It was left for general managers to re-code the report in their own terms. In this case the doctors used a management tool to argue for more resources and, since senior NHS managers granted this request, they presumably accepted that the budgetary case had indeed been made.

Although rarely touched on explicitly, the nature of rationing as rhetoric linked to micro-political struggles surfaces in many of the studies. Joyce points to the significance of managerialism and public health medicine in supporting a new economics-dominated discourse, which redefines the function of the health care system but also contributes to a 'fracturing' of governance at different levels of the system. The studies by Bourgeault and associates and Albrecht both point to the changing nature of *managed care*, influenced partly by increased pressure to cut costs within corporate medicine, and the growing tensions set up between administrators, professionals and patients. Lapsley and Melia, and Heritage and associates, document the continued power of medical professionals to blunt managerial initiatives that threaten to limit medical autonomy. Griffiths argues that 'gate keeping' and caseloads are a focus for conflict between psychiatrist managers and rank-and-file team members. In all these arenas we should expect to observe actors engaging in persuasive discourse in an attempt to ensure that resources are allocated in ways that suit their interests. There is typically what Geertz (1973: 316) terms a 'struggle for the real. The attempt to impose on the world a particular concept of how things at bottom are'. Increasingly claims and counter-claims about rationing feature explicitly in these exchanges.

The sociology of rationing remains an underdeveloped field, and the chapters in this volume make only a small – though we hope significant – contribution to changing that situation. It is a key arena for inter-disciplinary engagement and sociologists can play an important role in complementing and sometimes challenging the dominant economic perspective, which has framed many of the issues in a narrow and misleading way. Probably this new sub-field is best set within a wider sociology of resource allocation, which can draw on work from economic sociology, organisation studies and the sociology of health and illness to take back some of the territory that for too long has been conceded to other disciplines.

References

Aaron, H.J. and Schwartz, W.B. (1984) *The Painful Prescription: Rationing Health Care*. Washington, DC: Brookings Institute.

Begg, D., Fischer, S. and Dornbusch, R. (1987) *Economics*, 2nd Edition. London and New York: McGraw-Hill.

Boyd, E. (1998) Bureaucratic authority in the company of equals: the interactional management of medical peer review, *American Sociological Review*, 63, 200–224.

Byrd, D. E. (1981) *Organisational Constraints on Psychiatric Treatment: the Out-patient Clinic*. Greenwich, Connecticut: JAI Press.

Conrad, P. and Brown P. (1993) Rationing medical care: a sociological reflection, *Research in the Sociology of Health Care*, 10, 3–22.

Daniels, N. (1994) Meeting the challenges of justice and rationing. *Hastings Center Report*, 24, 4, 27–29.

Daniels, N., Light, D.W. and Caplan, R. (1996) *Benchmarks of Fairness for Health Care Reform*. New York: Oxford University Press.

Donaldson, C. (1996) Economics of priority setting: let's ration rationally! In Smith, R. (ed) *Rationing in Action*. London: BMJ Publishing Group.

Frader, J.E. and Bosk, C.E. (1981) Parent talk at intensive care unit rounds, *Social Science and Medicine*, 15E, 267–74.

Frankford, D.M. (1994) Scientism and economism in the regulation of health care, *Journal of Health Politics, Policy and Law*, 19, 158–9.

Freeman, V.G., Rathore, S.S., Weinfurt, K.P., Schulman, K.A. and Sulmasy, D.P. (1999) Lying for patients: physician deception of third-party payers, *Archives of Internal Medicine*, 159, 2263–70.

Geertz, C. (1973) *The Interpretation of Cultures*. New York: Basic Books.

Granovetter, M. (1985) Economic action and social structure: the problem of embeddedness, *American Journal of Sociology*, 91, 481–510.

Griffiths, L. and Hughes, D. (1994) 'Innocent parties' and 'disheartening' experiences: natural rhetorics in neuro-rehabilitation admissions conferences, *Qualitative Health Research*, 4, 385–410.

Griffiths, L. and Hughes, D. (1998) Purchasing in the British NHS: does contracting mean explicit rationing? *Health*, 2, 349–71.

Griffiths, L. and Hughes, D. (2000) 'Talking contracts and taking care: managers and professionals in the NHS internal market', *Social Science and Medicine*, 51, 209–222.

Hughes, D. and Griffiths, L. (1996) 'But if you look at the coronary anatomy...': risk and rationing in cardiac surgery, *Sociology of Health and Illness*, 18, 172–97.

Hughes, D. and Griffiths, L. (1997) 'Ruling in' and 'ruling out': two approaches to the micro-rationing of health care, *Social Science and Medicine*, 44, 589–99.

Hunter, D.J. (1997) *Desperately Seeking Solutions: Rationing Health Care*. London and New York: Longman.

Jeffrey, R. (1979) Normal rubbish: deviant patients in casualty departments, *Sociology of Health and Illness*, 1, 98–107.

Katz, M.J. and Rosen, H.S. (1991) *Microeconomics*. New York: Irwin.

Klein, R. (1990) From status to contract: the transformation of the British medical profession. In L'Etang, H. (ed) *Health Care Provision Under Constraints: a Decade of Change*. London: Royal Society of Medicine.

Lapsley, I. and Llewellyn, S. (1997) Statements of mutual faith: soft contracts in social care. In Flynn, R. and Williams, G. *Contracting for Health*. Oxford: Oxford University Press.

LeGrand, J. (1997) Knights, knaves or pawns? Human behaviour and social policy, *Journal of Social Policy*, 26, 149–69.

Light, D.W. (1980) *Becoming Psychiatrists: the Professional Transformation of Self*. New York: W.W. Norton.

Light, D.W. (1992) The practice and ethics of risk-rated health insurance, *Journal of the American Medical Association*, 267, 2503–8.

Light, D.W. (1997a) The restructuring of the American health care system. In Litman, T.J. and Robbins, L.S. (eds) *Health Politics and Policy*. Albany, NY: Delmar.

Light, D.W. (1997b) The real ethics of rationing, *British Medical Journal*, 315, 112–15.

Light, D.W. (2000) NHS waiting lists: the hidden agenda, *Consumer Policy Review*, 10, 4, 126–32.

Mechanic, D. (1995) Dilemmas in rationing health care services: the case for implicit rationing, *British Medical Journal*, 310, 1655–9.

Morreim, E.H. (1991) Gaming the system: dodging the rules, ruling the dodgers, *Archives of Internal Medicine*, 151: 443–7.

Redwood, H. (2000) *Why Ration Health Care?* Trowbridge: The Cromwell Press.

Reinhardt, U. (1996) *A Social Contract for 21st Century American Health Care: Three Tier Health Care with Bounty Hunting.* London: Nuffield Trust.

Roberts, C., Crosby, D., Grundy, P., Lewis, P., Long, J., Shellard, M. and Williams, A. (1996) The wasted millions, *The Health Service Journal*, 106, 5524, 24–7.

Roth, J.A. (1972) Some contingencies in the moral evaluation and control of clientele: the case of the hospital emergency service, *American Journal of Sociology*, 77, 839–57.

Spector, M. and Kitsuse, J. I. (1977) *Constructing Social Problems.* Menlo Park, California: Cummings.

Sudnow, D. (1965) Normal crimes: sociological features of the penal code in a public defender office, *Social Problems*, 12, 255–76.

Tannenbaum, S.J. (1994) Knowing and acting in medical practice, *Journal of Health Politics, Policy and Law*, 19, 27–44.

Wynia, M.K., Cummins, D.S., VanGeest, J.B. and Wilson, I.B. (2000) Physician manipulation of reimbursement rules for patients: between a rock and a hard place, *Journal of the American Medical Association*, 283, 1858–65.

Yates, J. (1996) *Private Eye, Heart and Hip: Surgical Consultants, the National Health Service and Private Medicine.* London: Churchill Livingstone.

2

Rationing through risk assessment in clinical genetics: all categories have wheels

Lindsay Prior

The web of medical technology

Lay understanding of the issues relating to human genetics has been extensively analysed in recent years (Durant *et al.* 1996, Kerr *et al.* 1998, Parsons and Atkinson 1992, Richards 1996). Using the results of such work, it is evident that everyday assessments of genetic inheritance are routinely tied into patterns of social (as well as biological) bonding (Richards 1997). For example, individuals very often interpret the amount of genetic material inherited from their relatives on the basis of facial resemblance or emotional 'closeness' rather than on the basis of Mendelian principles. And social factors, generally, tend to become embroiled in the assessment of genetic influences in a whole series of other ways.

This social grounding of lay thought is often contrasted with professional understanding of genetics. The latter is, of course, normally regarded as being driven by 'science' and scientific discovery – and thereby relatively uncontaminated by a consideration of social, political, or cultural factors. And it is certainly the case that within the rhetoric of scientific discussion, the assessment of inheritance patterns is regarded as an entirely objective and technical matter (Claus *et al.* 1991, McPherson *et al.* 1994).

I intend to focus on such technical assessments – especially in the context of risk calculations executed within a cancer genetics clinic. Risk calculations – of, say, the chances of any particular person inheriting a genetic abnormality – necessarily carry with them fundamental implications for patients and their doctors. Among these one would have to include the psychological wellbeing of patients, the implications for family interaction, the management of any potential therapies, the ethics of disclosure, the consequences for the insurability of affected relatives and much, much more. The British Medical Association's (BMA) human genetics group (1998), and the UK's House of Commons Select Committee (1995) have both outlined and reviewed a large number of the salient issues. In neither case, however, was rationing mentioned or dealt with as an inevitable consequence of the risk assessment process.

In what follows it is the interrelationships between assessments of genetic risk and policy issues relating to rationing that will be explored. In order to examine such connections, I have borrowed a guiding theme from work in the social construction of technology, and especially the work of Pinch and Bijker *et al.* (1989). The latter have indicated how technological processes, organisational procedures and social practices, such as those entailed by the use of modern clinical genetics, are routinely meshed together in a 'seamless web'. Such a position implies that one cannot regard the technology as standing isolated and divorced from social action – as inert tools merely to be used. Rather the concerns of various actors (say, clinicians, patients, laboratory scientists, support groups, administrators, politicians, and funding agencies) become interlocked in such a way that one has to comprehend the ensemble of practices and interests that make up the entire system, in order to understand how the technology is activated. Within that broader framework, problems concerning the manner in which specific technologies are recruited and 'translated' (Serres 1995: 159–63) loom large. Among the ensemble just spoken of are, of course, concerns relating to rationing. Rationing principles, however, are woven like a fine thread through the broad tapestry of action that takes place in the cancer genetics clinic, and the tracing of that thread requires, above all else, an examination of embedded practices.

Methodology and techniques of data collection

The data referred to in this chapter were derived from the study of a regional (UK) cancer genetics clinic. The clinic was initially established as a research clinic. During 1999 it was transformed into a National Health Service (NHS) facility, and just over 700 risk assessments were made on patients in the course of the calendar year. The clinic as a service also formed part of a much larger Institute that investigated and organised care relating to a wide variety of genetic conditions.

Data collected within the clinic/institute were of three kinds. First, there were data gathered from documents – from mission statements, referral criteria, research reports, anonymous family trees, clinical guidelines, and various (laboratory and computer generated) graphs and pictures associated with the assessment of genetic risk. Secondly, data were gathered from 'naturally occurring' organisational talk within the clinic/institute. Instances of such talk occurred in consultations between patients and professionals and between professionals themselves. For the purposes of this chapter detailed notes were taken on a small number of cancer genetic consultations (N = 4) held between patients and clinical staff. Thirdly, data were gathered from asking clinic professionals to explain and clarify risk assessment procedures. The professionals who were explicitly asked to explain such procedures were clinical geneticists (N = 4), nurse-counsellors (N = 2), and a laboratory scientist. The underlying principles of risk assessment, however, were sometimes best highlighted at seminars and research gatherings attended by other medical professionals – such as visiting scholars from other institutes and university-based primary care practitioners – and psychologists. During 1999–2000 six research meetings of various kinds were attended. Finally, a small number of formal (taped) interviews (N = 4) – specifically on the topic of rationing were conducted between the author and clinic professionals.

Interview and observation clearly have their place in social research, yet in a literate culture such as ours one of the most important of all available data sources is lodged within documents. Strangely – given the significance that writing plays in our culture – the role of documents in social research is widely underestimated (Prior 2001). Yet we know that routine scientific (and clinical) work is executed as much through writing as it is through conversation. Thus, Latour and Woolgar, in their study of the La Jolla laboratory, indicate how text can be as important as talk in scientific work, arguing, for example, that scientists are 'manic writers' (1979: 48). So scientists are constantly generating scientific facts through the use of written and other traces. Other traces – for example, charts and measures of all kind – being routinely derived from what Latour (1983) calls inscription devices. That is to say devices that turn material substances into documentary form. So one of Latour's injunctions for any research project is to 'look at the inscription devices' (1983: 161). The same kinds of thing can be said of work in clinics as of laboratories. In the site referred to in this chapter, people are of course talking about DNA, and 'mutations' rather than quasars, and the traces that they use are more likely to be radiographs, computer generated risk assessments, and sketches of family trees than physical trajectories. Nevertheless, we can say that genetic risk assessments are as much things that are inscribed – in various media – as they are talked about. Inevitably, then, a key point of focus for any researcher in the setting aforementioned has to be on how documents are used to assemble risks.

Although I have referred to naturally occurring talk and interview talk, the distinction is not, of course, as clear as it might seem from a distance (Potter 1997). For talk is always structured for some audience or other. Furthermore, using either kind of talk to generate what might be termed untarnished and unmediated data on the world external to the talk is highly problematic (Silverman 1993). In particular, it is evident that interview talk is not a source of independent and objective reports on the world, but rather a construction – often in narrative form – that is manufactured between interviewee and interviewer (Fontana and Frey 2000). Here, I have used the interviews as a mechanism for obtaining instigated 'accounts' about rationing (Radley and Billig 1996). Since rationing was a topic not ordinarily discussed within the clinic/institute, such accounts could only be derived from a formally structured interview process. The advantage of the interview material is that it generates data on issues that, in the day-to-day work of the clinic, were normally just taken for granted. The limitations of such data relate to the fact that such accounts were consciously and deliberately produced for the purpose of 'writing about rationing'. So there is a sense in which respondents were prompted to set into 'discursive consciousness' (Giddens 1984), issues that ordinarily remained part of 'practical consciousness'.

On a wider front, it might be thought that a study of just one clinic can tell us little about risk and rationing that is either representative or capable of generalisation. That would be a mistake for a number of reasons – not least because we know that the detailed study of single sites can generate some very useful results. Indeed, a focus on a single site such as the one mentioned herein, calls upon a strategy that has, over recent decades, generated some first class results in the sociology of science (Charlesworth et al. 1989, Knorr-Cetina 1983, Latour and Woolgar 1979, Lynch 1985). The latter work was, of course, executed in laboratories rather than clinics, but the principle is similar. And there are good grounds for arguing that, at the theoretical level, results based on a case study method are always generalisable. Indeed, those methodologists who advocate the use of the approach are keen to emphasise just how this is so. Thus Yin (1994), for example, points out how case studies produce results that are 'generalizable to theoretical propositions' rather than to populations or universes. Platt (1988), in her review of the method, points out that, whilst the method cannot tell us very much about the prevalence of particular characteristics in a community, it can offer a depth and richness of description and theoretical explanation that is indispensable to the social sciences. Further justification for case study analysis is contained in Ragin and Becker's (1992) edited collection. Abbott's (1992:62) claim therein, that by generating narratives of acting individuals rather than 'narratives of acting variables', case studies offer firmer grounds for policy analysis than do traditional modes of quantitative analysis is particularly pertinent. (See also, Stake 2000.) In short, then, the strength of case study research rests in the fact that it is situationally grounded.

As a number of authors have indicated (Klein et al. 1996, New and Le Grand 1996, Smith 1991), the rationing of health care resources is, more often than not, an implicit – almost secret – process. And many studies have shown how organisationally embedded social as well as clinical factors can affect medical decision making and resource allocation at ground level (Eisenberg 1979, Clark et al. 1991, Halper 1989, Hughes and Griffiths 1997). Given its implicit character, it is perhaps not so surprising that rationing was a topic that emerged only gradually out of the investigation that is reported on here. That is, it was something that appeared only after the researcher became engaged with the setting. In that sense the chapter might serve as an example as to how case study method can reveal topics and issues that would most likely remain hidden using research procedures that focused entirely on the investigation of pre-selected variables.

How is risk related to rationing?

'It is a truism to state that all health care systems ration care. The issue is not whether but how' (Hunter 1995: 877). And clearly, the 'how' of rationing can be unearthed at many different levels (Klein *et al.* 1996). Ham (1995: 825), for example, discerns five different levels at which priority-setting principles may be set. The range from the macro level of overall funding, through the allocation of funding for particular forms of treatment and care, down to decisions on how much to spend on individual patients. The focus in this chapter, however, is mainly on the fourth of Ham's five levels – the choice of which patients should receive access to treatment – and, only to a lesser extent on the last (how much to spend on individual patients).

Rationing (an organised process that restricts access to potentially beneficial, but scarce resources, by the application of a selection principle) is inexorably linked to risk assessment. Thus, when professionals judge people to be at 'high risk' of some disorder or other, they invariably seek to target scarce goods or facilities at the selected population. Such targeting is evident, for example, in UK programmes relating to the distribution of free influenza vaccine to those over 75 years of age, the immunisation of children against meningitis and in the provision of cancer screening services to women over 50. As a consequence of such targeting, a number of individuals in the 'low' or 'medium' risk groups who could benefit from such provision are normally excluded from access to it – purely on the basis of a population assessment. Indeed, rationing (in the sense above) is inevitable whenever population-based risk assessments are applied to individuals. This is irrespective of which country or health care system we choose to examine. In this chapter, of course, the focus is on cancer genetics, and it would probably be useful for me to sketch out how the allocation of an individual to a 'low', 'medium' or 'high' risk group might relate to the distribution of other (scarce, but potentially beneficial) resources. I shall use treatment decisions relating to breast cancer as an example.

Breast cancer, risk and rationing

Estimates of a breast cancer risk can impact on a number of treatment and management decisions. The most obvious of these would include admission to the genetics service itself. Women perceived to be at high and moderate risk ordinarily receive, if nothing else, expert advice and reassurance about their specific chances of succumbing to an inherited cancer. For example, it is known that breast cancer is an anxiety provoking issue for a large proportion of women, and family histories of the cancer are far from uncommon (Bortoff *et al.* 1996, Chalmers and Thompson 1996). As we shall see, however, a simple history of cancer in the family is far from sufficient for entry into the genetics service.

From the point of view of experts, and certainly as far as geneticists are concerned, being able to discriminate between those at high and those at low risk of a family-inherited cancer could be beneficial on a number of grounds. Screening issues are normally put at the top of the list of advantages. Thus, clinicians frequently mentioned, for example, how screening for colon cancers (the use of colonoscopy) was particularly beneficial for those at high risk, and how processes that were normally regarded by patients as unpleasant could be avoidable for low-risk individuals. In the realm of breast cancer it was the use of mammography that was referred to. Mammography is widely regarded as being effective for women aged 50–69 – it reduces breast cancer mortality by around one third (Kerlikowske et al. 1995). There is increasing evidence that it is useful for women aged between 40 and 49 (Feig 1997). In general, however, it is commonly held that the viability of mammography for women aged under 50 is limited. High rates of false positives are possible in younger women, together with the increased anxiety that such false positives generate. (In addition there is a potential for harm arising from exposure to radiation.) Furthermore, because rates of breast cancer are lower in women under 50 the cost of mammography per year of life saved rises. A recent US estimate, places this cost at around $100,000 (Salzman et al. 1997). Consequently, it has been argued that, at a population level, the high financial costs of a screening programme outweigh the clinical benefits (Wright et al. 1995).

A further set of considerations arises in relation to the use of post-menopausal hormone-replacement therapy (HRT). HRT is believed to increase the relative risk of breast cancer by some 30 to 40 per cent (Armstrong et al. 2000), whilst it halves the risk of coronary heart disease and osteoporosis. An ability to identify individuals at high-risk of breast cancer (say, according to a family history) could, therefore, have very important implications for the uptake of HRT in women aged over 50 years. (Note that the decision to opt for a therapy in relation to one condition has implications for the onset of other conditions, and so the resource implications of a given course of action are not always calculable.) Chemo-prevention might also enter into any cost-benefit equation. For example, Tamoxifen (a pharmaceutical treatment) may be used as a preventive measure (though not, currently, in Europe). And once again, apart from strict economic measures, one has to consider whether females who have been identified as being at a low or medium risk would benefit from such treatment. (In the US, the recommendation is that only women with a five year risk of breast cancer higher than 1.7 per cent should be prescribed Tamoxifen – Chlebowski et al. 1999). Finally, the possibility of prophylactic mastectomy has to be considered. A recent study estimated that for high-risk women prophylactic mastectomy could reduce the risk of breast cancer by 90 per cent (Hartmann et al. 1999). In the clinic to which this research refers, prophylactic mastectomy was mentioned by some women – with particularly marked family histories of breast cancer – as a first option.

Clearly, an expert decision as to whether such women were or were not high risk could have profound implications for their management programme.

Each of the possible therapeutic options has, then, costs and benefits for individual patients, their consultants and the public purse. Naturally, clinical geneticists were well aware of the issues. As one of the clinicians put it,

> CG1: You can see it [a risk category] affecting treatment decisions and quite expensive treatment decisions. And a perception of risk could be used [by a patient] either way, to affect the intensity of her treatment[1].

As I shall point out shortly, this is a statement replete with some rather important interpretations. For now, I wish to use it merely as a pointer to the fact that rationing in the sense of a restriction of supply, is a many-legged beast. Rationing, as selective targeting, can protect people from potentially harmful side effects of medical intervention, and can narrow down the population subjected to unpleasant procedures. (In that sense some parties might regard it as a positive and beneficial act.) It can also enable others to recruit their risk status so as to push for more treatment resources – as is hinted at in the above quotation. Furthermore, from the standpoint of health care funding agencies the close targeting of, say, high and moderate risk individuals in a screening programme could both reduce overall costs and reduce the cost per life saved. For reasons yet to be expounded upon, however, a process of rationing based on population-risk assessments can be detrimental to potentially large numbers of individuals.

Risk requires 'translation'

Risk looms large in contemporary medical discourse (Gabe 1995). Indeed, Skolbekken (1995) has spoken of a risk epidemic and has documented the marked rise of risk related publications during the 1967–91 period. So powerful has been the impact of risk analysis that Gifford (1986) has argued that risk has replaced cause as a focal point for clinical research. More recently, Førde (1998) has viewed such developments as an expression of a specific risk culture – a culture in part bolstered and fostered by epidemiology and public health sciences. Sciences that have been more concerned with aspects of probabilistic modelling than with microbiology per se. Whether that argument holds is not, of course, an issue that need be adjudicated on here. What is important to note is that risk and probability are intimately entwined. Indeed, those who adopt what is often referred to as the scientific position on risk claim that risk ought to be defined and assessed in terms of the concept of probability. Combined with this claim is another to the effect that scientific assessments of risk are both objective and factual in a way in which lay assessments are not. Thus, the (UK) Royal Society's 1992 document on risk states, 'A general concept of risk is the chance in quantitative terms, of a defined hazard occurring. It therefore combines a probabilistic measure of the occurrence of the primary event with a measure of the consequences of that/those event(s)' (1992: 4). This very distinctive, technocratic position on risk is further reiterated and buttressed in the Society's 1997 document, wherein it is stated that risk assessment is 'a purely technical matter involving calculations of the probabilities of harm based on the balance of available evidence' (1997: 46).

One problem with this line of argument is that 'probability' is a slippery concept. Indeed, within mathematics itself there are competing versions as to what 'probability' is (Hacking 1990). It is not appropriate to outline alternatives here. However, it is appropriate to state that one of the most persuasive of mathematical approaches is that which equates a probability to the frequency with which an event occurs in a long series of events (Prior *et al.* 2000) (for example, the frequency with which breast cancers are detected per year in a national population of females). Clearly, it is such population-based estimates of probability that epidemiologists use in their analyses of the rates with which particular forms of disease event (influenza, meningitis, lung cancer) appear. Yet, whilst epidemiologists derive their risk estimates from population assessments, clinicians deal only with individual cases. Inevitably, in the interstices between populations and individuals various difficulties can arise.

Let us assume, for example, that a group of clinicians use the probability of 0.25 as a cut-off point for some cancer screening service or other. By implication, such a policy will be detrimental to the small proportion of people whose chances of contracting a cancer are 1, but who are 'buried' in a sub-group that has a very low (population) prevalence – say, middle-aged males with breast cancer. This would be so, of course, no matter what the cut-off point were to be. For what the probability assessment is based on is a group, or a collective, and not an individual. Naturally, having derived a probability assessment from a collective, practitioners have necessarily to apply the assessment to individuals. The application of population-based assessments to individuals involves what we might call a translation – though it is not the only one. For, as Gifford (1986) indicates, a second translation occurs at the point where the clinician treats 'risk' as a pathology. That is, at the point when he or she identifies 'being-at-risk' as a clinically manageable condition. Both translations are evident in the work of the genetics clinic.

The backdrop to the clinical service

Recent scientific work in genetics has indicated that in some of the commoner cancers – breast, ovarian and colon – there is a Mendelian subset where genetic 'risk' is estimated to be high, but which cannot be clearly distinguished on clinical or pathological grounds from other cancers. (However, methods – gene expression methods – are currently being developed to overcome this difficulty.) In the case of ovarian, breast and colorectal cancer the subsets can be identified by the use of molecular tests. For example, the two genes associated with breast cancer (BRCA1 and 2 – located on chromosomes 17q and 13q respectively) are believed to be carried by around 1.7 per thousand people – though they are probably responsible for only some five per cent of all breast cancers (Department of Health 1998). BRCA1 is also associated with ovarian cancer. The incidence of cancer with a familial predisposition as a whole is probably in the region of one in 30 individuals – so about 10 per cent of all cancers have a familial subgroup (McPherson *et al.* 1994). The penetrance of some of these genes is estimated to be as high as 0.8 – implying that an individual possessing the mutation is at a very high mathematical risk of succumbing to cancer.

The clinical service that forms the focus for this chapter was established during the late 1990s – partly in response to the aforementioned discoveries. It was designed in line with the principles referred to in the Calman-Hine Report on cancer services (Department of Health 1995), and the 1998 Working Group on Genetics and Cancer Services (Department of Health 1998). The clinic offers a service to those who are referred to it by GPs and secondary care specialists. It includes: risk assessment (on the basis of family history), counselling and advice giving, predictive genetic testing for well women and men at risk of cancer; the organisation of presymptomatic surveillance for those at increased risk; information packages and specialised nursing support; and education and training of health professionals. During 1999 there were some 703 referrals to the service.

Rationing principles appear at various points in the service. The most obvious juncture, however, is that concerned with admission into the service itself. For, as I have already pointed out, although many families can demonstrate a 'history' of cancers the decision as to whether such histories are or are not significant is a matter left to expert geneticists.

Risk categories have wheels

Currently, there are no commonly agreed standards (either in the UK or elsewhere) for deciding when an individual falls into a prima facie category of high risk. In some services, referrals to genetics clinics are idiosyncratic. For that reason the regional clinic referred to here adopted, and recently circulated, a list of eligibility or inclusion criteria – designed to standardise referrals. For example, as far as breast cancer is concerned, inclusion requires at least one of the following criteria to be met. One first-degree female aged under 40 affected; two first-degree relatives (on the same side of the family) affected at 60 years of age or less, three first- or second-degree relatives of any age (on the same side of the family); one first-degree female with bilateral breast cancer; one first-degree male breast cancer. Different criteria (the Amsterdam criteria) would be used for colorectal cancers (see Vasen *et al*. 1991). For ovarian cancers the requirement would be for two or more such cancers within the family with at least one first-degree relative affected. (A first-degree relative would be a parent or a sibling.)

How such criteria are actually used by those who refer people to the clinic is not at all clear. What is important from our standpoint, however, is that the boundaries between high and low risk implied by the criteria are malleable. So it would be possible, for example, for the clinical service to alter the above filtering rules so as to abolish, say, the age barrier of 40 in the first-degree relative, or to alter the requirement for three first-degree relatives at any age, to two such relatives. The criteria are certainly not set in concrete, and as such they may be seen as arbitrary.

SOC: The category high risk is movable isn't it? It seems to me as a lay person that all the categories are on wheels.

CG1:   Oh. Absolutely.

Naturally, this raises the issue as to how such wheels come to rest where they do. At first it might be thought that the division between high-, medium-, and low-risk categorisations would be determined by 'the science'. Indeed, there are numerous guidelines for who and who should not be allocated to the various categories (Pharoah *et al*. 1998, Eccles *et al*. 2000). And such guidelines are normally presented as objective – taking into account only who might benefit from the categorisations. Yet, as the following interview extract, demonstrates, 'science' is always embedded in a set of organised social practices. So, for example, in designing the filters for the service one has to be mindful of the consequent volume of demand. Indeed, one of the most important considerations for specifying referral criteria in a clinic such as this concern the availability of resources in general.

SOC: So, depending on how you specify the cut-off points, it has implications for resources. Yes?

CG1:   I always thought it worked the other way around. That you decided how many people you could cope with in terms of service provision, or what would be appropriate for those at high risk, and set your risk figures so that you got just about the right number of people coming through for your service.

Thus, the 'web' that was referred to in the opening section is one that embraces far more then what might be considered to be straightforward clinical or scientific criteria. In the above instance, 'resources' seem to come first. Indeed, as sociologists of science and technology such as Latour

(1987), and Bijker *et al.* (1989) have indicated, the pursuit of scientific (or clinical) work invariably involves a consideration of various issues. Hence, professional scientists have always to assemble coalitions – of things, people, and interests – in order to activate their technologies. What is more, such acts of assemblage are not peripheral to science, but rather at its core. It is not perhaps so surprising, then, that all the clinic professionals made some degree of reference to what might be conventionally considered as 'extra-scientific' or extra-clinical factors.

> CG2: It's a question where do you put the boundaries in terms of what you call high risk and what you call low risk and what you call intermediate. You can shift them around. And we have actually often put the thing completely back to front along the lines that, OK, maybe high risk and maybe not so high, but we have been given so much money to sort it out and given that we have only got so much money: that means that if you are going to put it in particular directions you have to set a cut-off point. So, if you are given only a small amount of money, then, OK, then maybe you are only going to be able to sort out a small number of very high-risk people and provide a service for them. If you were to give us a bit more then we could move the cut-off point along a bit and [so on].

Informant CG4 had originally argued that the cut-off points had been selected on the basis of 'research interests' alone (any woman with a risk of 0.5 or higher being accepted into the clinic). However, he too made mention of a broader web especially as the clinic was now dealing with a vastly increased number of patients at exactly the same funding as was received when the clinic was in its research phase. Hence,

> CG4: We have an issue to grapple with which is, how will we continue to test/
> SOC: /at the molecular level?
> CG4:   /at the molecular level when the client population is increasing? We haven't got a resolution to that at the moment....
> SOC: Is it likely that you will have to move up the 50 per cent cut-off point?
> CG4: We have two options don't we? [We can both maintain the cut-off point and receive more funding or], the alternative is that we would have to alter the threshold at which we offer testing.
> SOC: And by implication the definition of high risk/
> CG4:   /The definition of high-risk would change, so people who previously would have got testing will not get testing..

In short, then, being at high risk is a matter determined by reference to a web of concerns. Among such concerns are those relating to financial resources. One might even argue that, in this service, it is the latter that shaped the nature of the risk categories. In that respect it might be thought that the chapter highlights an issue peculiar to health care systems in which there are limited budgets, but that would be a mistake. For, in the way of the world, resources are always finite. Thus Heidmal *et al.* (1999) in their discussion of a Norwegian clinical service point toward restrictions that arise as a result of there being a limited number of skilled counsellors able to deal with those identified as being 'at risk' of breast cancer. So finance is not always a key constraint. Indeed, the sociological point is that the activation of science, technology, and medicine never occur in some pure state – untainted by social, economic, ideational or cultural contexts and resources. The web is omnipresent, though its exact shape and the precise components within it are always open to empirical inquiry. Just to emphasise how that was so, I shall end this section with further reference to the influence of what would normally be called 'extra-scientific' factors;

CG3:   We tried to extrapolate from what was proving to be the experience in regions which had rushed in and were offering a [genetics] service ... and seeing a huge expansion in the numbers of referrals and were clearly going to be swamped. And, er/

SOC: /And that's because their threshold points were too low do you think?

CG3:   Well. I don't. I don't. I don't. Well. It sounds a bit smug, but I don't think that they had thought it through properly. Or they could argue that had a different approach which was to offer what they thought what was an appropriate service and then clamour for extra funding when their resources were clearly inadequate. That would be another way of going about it.

Designing risk categories and their associated cut-off points is clearly, then, a matter that involves a consideration of resources. The formulation of such categories is, nevertheless, only part of the risk assessment process. More important from the standpoint of an individual patient is allocation to one or other of the categories themselves. Yet, there too, 'science' is affected by context.

Risk is fashioned by inscription devices

To determine the risk status of individuals, the personnel of the clinic sought two types of evidence. The first related to a family history and the second to the results of molecular tests.

Family history is derived from a questionnaire that is dispatched to the patient at the point of referral. On return of the questionnaire a telephone interview about that family history is conducted by the genetics nurse/ counsellor. Where suspicion of inherited breast cancer is involved, a risk calculation is subsequently made based on the information received. This is partly achieved through the use of a programme known as CYRILLIC. Thus, on receipt of the answers to the aforementioned questionnaire, the family history data are normally fed into CYRILLIC (Chapman 1997). CYRILLIC produces a family tree together with a numerical risk estimate. Based on the information generated, an assessment of the case is then made at a weekly meeting of the consultant and the nurse/counsellors. Referrals can be classified as 'low', 'medium' or 'high risk'. A person considered to be at low risk is referred back to his or her GP for further advice and reassurance. A person deemed to be at moderate risk is also referred back to his or her GP, or consultant, with a covering letter referring to screening needs or other interventions. The nurse/counsellor may also contact the patient by phone so as to explain the nature of the risk assessment. Only those who fall clearly within the high-risk category are invited to attend the genetics clinic for further assessment and involvement in the full array of clinical procedures – counselling, screening, and testing.

In line with what has been stated above, estimates of being at risk of breast (or of any other) cancer is commonly calculated as an average lifetime risk (currently around one in eight for female breast cancer). But for any individual the risk may be higher or lower. Indeed, risk alters according to such things as age, age at menarche and so on – thus a 50-year-old woman who has not had breast cancer has a lifetime risk of 11 per cent instead of 12 per cent. In that sense a risk is flexible.

SOC: Your risk isn't fixed is it? For breast cancer?
CG2: No. And [a change of calculation] will sometimes put you into a different risk management category.

In the realm of genetics, risk estimates are commonly calculated according to particular statistical models – such as the Gail model (Spiegelman et al. 1994) or the Claus model (Claus et al. 1996). The role of family history – and of other factors – is somewhat different in each model and so a given woman's risk of cancer is dependent not simply on items drawn from her personal biography, but also on the relative weight that is given to different factors. Not surprisingly, therefore, in a recent comparison of risk assessments applied to 200 UK women attending a breast cancer clinic (Tischkowitz et al. 2000), it was noted that the proportion of such women allocated to a high risk (of hereditary breast cancer) category varied markedly – from 0.27 using one method, as against 0.53 for a second method. A third method allocated only 0.14 to the high-risk category. So there are some women for whom risk is systematically 'underestimated' by the very nature of the models. This is so because the populations on which the risk models are based are themselves biased. For example, they contain only (North American) women; women who predominantly work in the professions, and women with documented family histories. Further, the samples under-represent ethnic groups known to be at high risk – such as women of Ashkenazi Jewish descent.

Such biases in the computerised inscription devices naturally create difficulties for clinicians. They are, however, difficulties that in many ways serve only to underline the problems inherent in the primary translation of risk previously mentioned. For, as the following interview extracts demonstrate, the clinical focus is on persons rather than populations, and personal histories frequently fail to match up to the standards contained in the inscription devices.

CG1: The person that they [the models] don't do any favours to I suppose, or don't allow you to assess really, is the sort of woman who has had a great grandmother with breast cancer aged 35, and then its come down the male line and there's been no women around. And she just wouldn't qualify for anything ...

SOC: So the extent to which a woman can be given a risk figure does depend on the number of close female relatives?

CG: Y:Yes.

The reference to the 'male line', then, emphasises the gender bias in the aforementioned devices. And, the following extract highlights how people with a lack of a documented history fall outside device competence.

CG2: In any low-risk group you are going to have a few people who really are at high risk, but you don't know it.

SOC: Because the family history doesn't suggest any abnormality?

CG2: Sure. And they may not have much family. Their mothers might have died young from something else and the brothers don't show anything.

An example as to how a risk assessment for one and the same person alters according to the statistical model being used is provided in Figure 1. (Risk calculations are based not simply on family history but also the history of the index case who in this instance had no children, no breast biopsies and an age at menarche of 15.)

When risk prediction models indicate a person as falling within the high-risk category then the possibility of genetic susceptibility testing arises. That is to say, it becomes feasible to consider the use of blood samples and subsequent laboratory analysis to determine the presence of mutations. In the case of breast cancer it is estimated that the presence of BRCA1 and 2 suggest a lifetime risk of such cancer to be within the range of 60–85 per cent, and risk of ovarian cancer of about 15–40 per cent (Armstrong et al. 2000). A woman belonging to a high-risk family where no mutation is

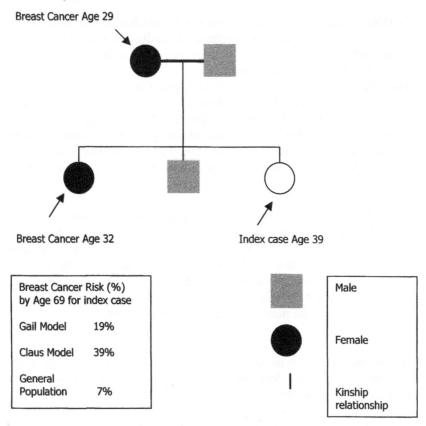

Figure 1. *Risk estimates from two breast cancer assessment models*

detected would, of course, require a different risk assessment – though there are currently no models available for adjusting the prediction. As with the risk mathematics referred to above, however, laboratory evidence can be generated in a variety of ways and is always in need of interpretation. For example, the fact that the BRCA1 mutation is not evident on the radiograph (yet another example of a Latourian inscription device) does not necessarily mean that the individual is at low risk. In that light it is also of interest to note that even when the laboratory evidence shows the presence of an abnormality, expert knowledge is required to determine whether it is or is not 'relevant'.

SOC: As far as spotting mutations are concerned, will any change in a [gene] sequence do?

CG4: There are some changes that regularly crop up in families with a lot of breast cancer. There are other changes that might be unique to that family and which you think probably don't have any effect on the protein made by that gene and therefore probably irrelevant. But there can be room for uncertainty of that. ... If it doesn't alter the amino acid sequence in the protein then you think it probably will not be harmful.

So estimates of risk can be altered at any of the relevant stages: at the referral stage, at the family history stage, or, indeed, at the stage of molecular investigation. A statistical risk is neither fixed nor easily determined, but rather assembled through a series of social practices.

The limitations of technology

I have referred to two translations – of population data into personal risk, and of 'risk' into pathology[2]. Both translations permeate the daily work of the clinic. Thus,

CG4: Partly it is our clinical experience over the last few years. The [statistical] models we know are flawed. We don't take the models other than as a guide. And I think that that is really important [... and] I do worry about whether or not we can build in appreciation about all the errors that are inevitable in population based data that was used to generate those models. So, for example, I saw a family yesterday. [The nurse/counsellor] had the pedigree and we put it into this computer programme and it came up with a lower risk than we expected. It didn't give a high-risk result. And yet when you looked at the family tree clinically, the reason for that was that the breast cancer was close but there was an intervening male, ... and it was on her Dad's side of the family. And as we discussed earlier the models aren't used to that. And yet there was a huge family history but because this man was in between the model isn't flexible enough to interpret that. And my worry is that if that women had gone to one of the 10 [WWW] sites or models that one can plug one's own details into, those models would have given her a low risk.

As we have seen (Figure,1) it is possible to get a different risk estimate for one and the same person by using a different programme. (However, the clinicians believed that their referral criteria would always pick up people with at least three times the population risk.) In relation to a suspected mutation for colorectal cancers, computer calculations of risk are unavailable, and so categorisation into the low- and high-risk bands is achieved on the basis of family history alone. This means that there is considerable room for the application of expert judgement in arriving at any risk assessment.

Indeed, in the present study geneticists were keen to indicate how essential access to this expert advice actually is. They normally made reference to it in the context of patients being able to buy into genetic testing through commercial firms such as Myriad Genetics. And they argued that negative findings on the molecular test did not necessarily mean that a person was at population (average) risk – for only a detailed family history plus molecular evidence could suggest that. This was especially so in relation to colorectal cancer where it was pointed out that over one third of patients with a distinct family history of Hereditary Non Polyposis Colorectal Cancer (HNPCC) showed no evidence of any abnormality in the DNA sequence.

This method of using a family history as a gateway to the search for mutations is of interest to us for a number of reasons. First, it enables geneticists to exert some degree of professional control over who is and who is not eligible for genetic testing. Secondly, it creates a space in which counselling and advice sessions might be directed toward those who need them. (The clinicians were always keen to indicate that this was not provided by commercial testing agencies.) Thirdly, it is, in many ways, more resource efficient than a process that channels the patient directly into the molecular testing phase[3] – and this is not merely because it focuses only on a pre-defined high risk group. For searching for mutations in BRCA1 or BRCA2 is a complex process (Rosenblatt *et al.* 1996). The genes involved are long sequences. Abnormalities of some kind or another are always present, and the identification of harmful mutations in clinic samples had sometimes taken up to 12 months to identify. In some cases abnormalities were never found.

Recruiting risk to ask for more

CG2: The way things actually work in practice is that people that shout loudest or people who have got sort of enthusiastic backers, or who are articulate or whatever, they are the ones that end up getting the money spent on them. And it's not very often that you have a plan that can actually be worked out, because you are usually reacting...

Despite its shadowy nature, it is clear that rationing implies planning. And however flawed a rationing principle may be when examined in the framework of social justice, it will at least serve to operate as a distribution mechanism for the scarce resources at hand. Yet, whether it be just or unjust, it is always possible to subvert rationing principles. They can be subverted by other professionals (as is suggested in the above quotation), and/or by patients themselves. Indeed, it is clear that rationing principles can be used by different parties for various ends, and that there is a dynamic to rationing that is rarely referred to in the literature.

Patients, of course, are normally viewed as passive recipients of rationing. Yet, in the clinic in which this work was undertaken there seemed to be an awareness that patients were well capable of recruiting their risk status to squeeze more from 'the system'. Such claims were usually mentioned in relation to the identification of early-onset (childhood) or reproductive disorders rather than late-onset disorders such as cancers. And the systems that were supposedly squeezed related to education or social services provision rather than health service resources. Whether parents did in fact use the 'at risk' status of their children to ask for more was a matter that lay beyond the boundaries of this investigation, but it did raise the interesting issue of how 'cancer' patients might recruit risk in their everyday lives. This notion of using a risk status to ask for more is only one facet of recruitment, of course. For it is also possible for individuals to use their risk status as a building block of personal identity. Such integration of risk into identity has been well documented for HIV/AIDS patients (Green and Sobo 2000).

In the context of use, the most pertinent issues arise out of the possibility for testing for mutations by commercial agencies[4]. Commercial testing for abnormalities is already available. For reasons that I have indicated, however, whether someone is at a high or low risk of succumbing to a disorder is a matter for qualitative judgement. Thus, there is, for example, a degree of uncertainty over which kinds of alterations in the genetic template might be causative. 'Redundancy' or interchange in the CAGT sequences of the DNA is, in a sense, in-built into the process and requires expert interpretation. Lay interpretations of what is or is not a significant change in the sequence may, however, differ from expert assessments. The lay 'landscape of risk' (Green and Sobo 2000), looks different from the landscape of the professionals. Where numerical assessments are involved, lay cut-off points for high risk are unlikely to match professional ones. So the possibility arises of the more affluent members of the population seeking out commercially available information on their risk status and using the results to turn risk into need – to demand or acquire more frequent screening, prophylactic measures or even extensive counselling facilities. Risk assessment in that light can be seen as a many-edged sword. It is, of course, not at all clear how lay people will use information about abnormalities in the genetic sequence. I shall end this section with a reference to the fears of CG4. He is discussing the possible consequences of ready access to commercial testing.

CG4: There's no commitment [on behalf of the companies that test] for interpreting that result. And effectively I believe that we will end up with a huge number of people that will be falsely re-assured by this testing. And a small, but increasing number of people that will be acutely anxious with no prior counselling, who will come hammering on the door. I don't think that they will be knocking [as SOC had suggested]. They will be kicking the door down. And it will completely overwhelm or subvert a structure that we have in place.

Conclusion

Maynard argues that rationing in the health care sector involves who will be given '"right" of access to care and who, as a result of denial, will be left in pain and discomfort, and, in the limit, to die' (1995: 5). In the light of this study, that seems to present a rather blunt and very crude notion of what rationing can involve.

The focus herein has been on genetic risk assessment and its relationship to rationing. In such a context, it is clear that the amount and kinds of resources allocated to 'at risk' individuals are very much dependent on how a person is classified in terms of a risk category. So, the flow of advice relating to counselling services, screening, prophylactic surgery and medical treatment are all linked to the risk-assessment process. Yet, we have also noted how evaluations of risk as 'high', 'medium' and 'low' are judgements that are composed on a the basis of several considerations – mathematical considerations being, on occasion, the least significant. As a result, the boundaries between risk categories are movable. That is to say, the decision to create a cut-off point between medium- and high-risk individuals (for any given condition) – at, say, four affected relatives rather than three – is, in many ways, arbitrary. For example, in the service that is referred to in this chapter, considerations of 'demand' and 'resources' loomed large. Consequently, the high-risk criteria were set so as to net around 10 high-risk families per million of the population. In other settings a rather different web of influences may operate. What such influences may be can only be discovered empirically, for risk and rationing involve processes that are situated. In that light it is grounded investigations, rather than broad-brush pronouncements of the relevant issues, that are required.

As far as social studies of risk are concerned, this accords exactly with recent calls for research to be organisationally contextualised (Horlick-Jones 2000). In our case study we have not only noted how risk is assembled according to a mélange of social, economic and scientific interests, but also how risk requires translation – as Gifford (1986) has argued. On a broader front, the case study has also revealed how medical technology is necessarily activated within a social, cultural and political web in such a way that it is ensembles of practices that need to be studied rather than isolated applications of technique. To think in terms of a strict division between science and technology, and the social is, in that sense, erroneous.

As well as demonstrating how rationing is embedded in routine organisational activities, this study has also highlighted how rationing decisions are open to manipulation by various parties. Rationing is not – as Maynard (1999) would have it – simply a top-down managerial process in which health care administrators deny resources to those in need. Thus, we ended by suggesting how risk categories may be recruited by both professionals and lay people to organise the distribution of scarce resources in line with their own concerns.

Above all, we have seen how rationing is the process that dare not speak its name. In fact, it is not a term that is readily used within the environs of the clinic. Hence, in the day-to-day work of the institute it is discourses of 'risk' that are called upon to justify resource distribution. In that sense the language of risk serves to mask the all-pervasive process of rationing.

During recent decades the sociology of clinical encounters has tended to concentrate on the study of doctor-patient interaction and issues of communication. In particular, there has been a tendency to examine and analyse the entities and phenomena that patients and physicians, as actors, bring into the clinic. In that respect the relevant points of sociological focus have been on such things as the body, the illness, disability, and disease – and the manner in which they are assembled and interpreted through episodes of interaction. A focus on what we might call the background organisational procedures in terms of which clinical encounters are framed has been less evident. Yet, it is clear, in so many ways, that who the 'patient' is, and what pathology and risk they carry are all features that are allocated through organisational processes that pre-structure any particular clinical episode. So, for example, modern genetics necessarily takes the family (rather than any individual) as the patient, and identifies pathologies and risks by analysing family pedigrees, rather than the anatomy of the isolated individual. One might say that patients, risks, bodies and their pathology are shaped by organisational priorities. In that context one is tempted to argue that there is always far more in heaven and earth (and medical clinics) than interaction and the exchange of interpersonal communications. A focus on rationing, at the very least, serves to underline the significance of such organisational features in routine clinical work, and, consequently, to set organisational procedures centre-stage.

Acknowledgements

The work reported on was preliminary to the execution of research funded by the ESRC under the Innovative Health Technologies Programme (Award L218252046). I would like to record my thanks to ESRC for the award, and to the professionals who worked in the study clinic. Any faults or shortcomings in the analysis are, of course, entirely mine. Thanks are also due to an anonymous reviewer, and to the editors, for constructive criticism on earlier drafts of this chapter.

Notes

1 In the following extracts CG = Clinical Geneticist. SOC = the researcher.
2 In response to this point, one of the clinicians argued that this is necessarily the case since there is never any sharp line to be drawn between having and not having a cancer. Getting cancer is a multi-step event. Pathology (such as a constitutional mutation in a tumour-suppressor gene) can be present even before cancer can be detected under the pathologist's microscope.

3   The average cost of DNA extraction + production of an aliquot by PCR + Heteroduplex Analysis + a Protein Truncation Test at the clinic was £98. Confirmation of any mismatches brought that cost to around £234 per sample. These tests only look at a proportion of the BRCA1 and BRCA2 genes. Myriad Genetics offers a sequencing test (in a very short turn-around time) at a cost of around $2400.
4   See, for example, http://www.myriad.com/

References

Abbott, A. (1992) What do cases do? Some notes on activity in sociological analysis. In Ragin, C.C. and Becker, H.S. (eds) *What is a Case? Exploring the foundations of social inquiry*. Cambridge: Cambridge University Press.

Armstrong, K., Essen, A. and Weber, B. (2000) Assessing the risk of breast cancer, *The New England Journal of Medicine*, 342, 8, 564–71.

Bijker, W.E., Hughes, T.P. and Pinch, T. (eds) (1989) *The Social Construction of Technological Systems*. Cambridge, MA: MIT Press.

Bortoff, J.L., Ratner, P.A., Johnson, J.L. *et al.* (1996) Uncertainties and challenges. Communicating risk in the context of familial cancer. *Report to the National Cancer Institute of Canada*. Vancouver, BC: Institute of Health Promotion Research. University of British Columbia.

British Medical Association (1998) *Human Genetics. Choice and Responsibility*. Oxford: Oxford University Press.

Chalmers, K. and Thomson, K. (1996) Coming to terms with the risk of breast cancer: perceptions of women with primary relatives with breast cancer, *Qualitative Health Research*, 6, 2, 256–82.

Chapman, C.J. (1997) *Cyrillic for Pedigree Drawing*. Cherwell Scientific Publishing.

Charlesworth, M., Farrall, L., Stokes, T. and Turnbull, D. (1989) *Life Among the Scientists. An Anthropological study of an Australian Scientific Community*. Melbourne: Oxford University Press.

Chlebowski, R.T. Collyar, D.E., Somerfield, M.R. and Pfister, D.G. (1999) American Society of Clinical Oncology technology assessment on breast cancer risk reduction strategies: tamoxifene and raloxifene, *Journal of Clinical Oncology*, 17, 1939–55.

Claus, E.B., Risch, N. and Thompson, W.D. (1991) Genetic analysis of breast cancer in the cancer and steroid hormone study, *American Journal of Human Genetics*, 48, 232–42.

Clark, A.C., Potter, D.A. and McKinlay, J.B. (1991) Bringing social structure back into clinical decision making, *Social Science and Medicine*, 32, 853–66.

Department of Health (1995) A policy framework for commissioning cancer services. *A Report by the Expert Advisory Group on Cancer to the Chief Medical Officer of England and Wales*. London: Department of Health and Welsh Office.

Department of Health (1998) *Genetics and Cancer Services. Report of a Working Group*. London: Department of Health.

Durant, J., Hansen, A. and Bauer, M. (1996) Public understanding of the new genetics. In Marteau, T. and Richards, M. (eds) *The Troubled Helix: Social and Psychological Implications of the New Genetics*. Cambridge: Cambridge University Press.

Eccles, D.M., Evans, D.G.R. and Mackay, J. (2000) Guidelines for a genetic risk based approach to advising women with a family history of breast cancer, *Journal of Medical Genetics*, 37, 203–9.

Eisenberg, J.M. (1979) Sociologic influences on decision making by clinicians, *Annals of Internal Medicine,* 90, 957–64.

Feig, S.A. (1997) Increased benefit from shorter screening mammography intervals for women aged 40-49 years, *Cancer*, 80, 2035–9.

Fontana, A. and Frey, J.H. (2000) The Interview. From structured questions to negotiated text. In Denzin, N.K. and Lincoln, Y.S. (eds.), *Handbook of Qualitative Research*. 2nd. Edition. London: Sage.

Førde, O.H. (1998) Is imposing risk awareness cultural imperialism? *Social Science and Medicine*, 47, 9, 1155–9.

Gabe, J. (ed) (1995) *Medicine, Health and Risk. Sociological Approaches*. Oxford: Blackwell.

Giddens, A. (1984) *The Constitution of Society*. Cambridge: Polity Press.

Gifford, S.M. (1986) The meaning of lumps. A case study of the ambiguities of risk. In Janes, C.R., Stall, R. and Gifford, S.M. (eds) *Anthropology and Epidemiology*. Dordrecht: D.Reidel.

Green, G. and Sobo, E.J. (2000) *The Endangered Self. Managing the Social Risks of HIV*. London Routledge.

Hacking, I. (1990) *The Taming of Chance*. Cambridge: Cambridge University Press.

Halper, T. (1989) *The Misfortunes of Others. End-stage Renal Disease in the UK*. Cambridge: Cambridge University Press.

Ham, C. (1995) Synthesis: what can we learn from international experience? *Medical Bulletin*, 51, 819-30.

Hartmann L.C., Schaid, D.J., Woods, J.E. *et al.* (1999) Efficacy of bilateral prophylactic mastectomy in women with a family history of breast cancer, *New England Journal of Medicine*, 340,77–84.

Heidmal, K., Maehle, L. and Møller, P. (1999) Costs and benefits of diagnosing familial breast cancer, *Disease Markers*, 15, 1–3, 167–73.

Horlick-Jones, T. (2000) Towards a new risk analysis? *ESRC. Risk and Human Behaviour Newsletter*, Number 8, 7–13.

House of Commons Science and Technology Committee (1995) *Third Report. Human Genetics: The Science and its Consequences*. London: HMSO.

Hughes, D. and Griffiths, L. (1997) 'Ruling in' and 'ruling out': two approaches to the micro-rationing of health care, *Social Science and Medicine*, 44, 589–99.

Hunter, D. J. (1995) Rationing health care. The political perspective, *Medical Bulletin*, 51, 876–84.

Kerlikowske, K., Grady, D., Rubin, S.M., Sandrock, C. and Ernster, V.L. (1995) Efficacy of screening mammography: a meta-analysis, *Journal of the American Medical Association*, 273, 149–54.

Kerr, A., Cunningham-Burley, S. and Amos, A. (1998) Drawing the line: an analysis of lay people's discussions about the new genetics, *Public Understanding of Science*, 7, 113–33.18.

Klein, R., Day, P. and Redmaybe, S. (1996) *Managing Scarcity*. Buckingham: Open University Press.

Knorr-Cetina, K. (1983) The ethnographic study of scientific work: toward a constructivist interpretation of science. In Knorr-Cetina, K.D. and Mulkay, M. (eds) *Science Observed*. London: Sage.

Latour, B. (1983) Give me a laboratory and I will raise the world. In Knorr-Cetina, K.D. and Mulkay, M. (eds) *Science Observed*. London: Sage.

Latour, B. (1987) *Science in Action. How to follow Engineers in Society*. Milton Keynes: Open University Press.

Latour, B. and Woolgar, S. (1979) *Laboratory Life. The Social Construction of Scientific Facts*. London: Sage Publications.

Lynch, M. (1985) *Art and Artifact in Laboratory Science. A Study of Shop Work and Shop Talk in a Research Laboratory*. London: Routledge and Kegan Paul.

Maynard, A. (1999) Rationing health care: an exploration, *Health Policy*, 49, 5–11.

McPherson, K., Steel, C.M. and Dixon, J.M. (1994) Breast cancer – epidemiology, risk factors and genetics, *British Medical Journal*, 309, 1003–6.

New, B. and Le Grand, J. (1996) *Rationing in the NHS: Principles and Pragmatism*. London: King's Fund.

Parsons, E. and Atkinson, P. (1992) Lay constructions of genetic risk, *Sociology of Health and Illness*, 1, 437–55.

Pharoah, P.D., Stratton, J. F. and Mackay, J. (1998). Screening for breast and ovarian cancer: the relevance of family history, *British Medical Bulletin*, 54, 823-38.

Pinch, T.J. and Bijker, W.E. (1989) The social construction of facts and artifacts: or how the sociology of science and the sociology of technology might benefit each other. In Bijker, W.E., Hughes, T.P. and Pinch, T. (eds) *The Social Construction of Technological Systems*. Cambridge, Ma: MIT Press.

Platt, J. (1988) What can case studies do?. In Burgess, R. (ed) *Studies in Qualitative Methodology*. Volume 1. Stamford CT: JAI Press.

Potter, J. (1997) Discourse analysis as a way of analysing naturally occurring talk. In Silverman, D. (ed) *Qualitative Research. Theory, Method and Practice*. London: Sage.

Prior, L. (2001) *Using Documents in Social Research*. London: Sage. (In press)

Prior, L., Glasner, P. and McNally, R. (2000) Genotechnology: three challenges to risk legitimation. In Adam, B., Beck, U. and Van Loon, J. (2000) *The Risk Society and Beyond*. London: Sage.

Radley, A. and Billig, M. (1996) Accounts of health and illness: dilemmas and representations, *Sociology of Health and Illness*, 18, 2, 220–40.

Ragin, C. C. and Becker, H.S. (eds) (1992) *What is a Case? Exploring the Foundations of Social Inquiry*. Cambridge: Cambridge University Press.

Richards, M. (1996) Lay and professional knowledge of genetics and inheritance, *Public Understanding of Science*, 5, 217–30.

Richards, M. (1997) It runs in the family. lay knowledge about inheritance. In Clarke, A. and Parsons, E. (eds) *Culture, Kinship and Genes. Towards Cross-Cultural Genetics*. Basingstoke: Macmillan.

Rosenblatt, D.S., Foulkes, W.D. and Narod, S.A. (1996) Genetic Screening for Breast Cancer, *New England Journal of Medicine*, 334, 18, 1201.

Royal Society (1992) *Risk. Analysis, Perception and Management*. London. The Royal Society.

Royal Society (1997) *Science, Policy and Risk*. London: Royal Society.

Saltzman, P., Kerlikowske, K. and Phillips, K. (1997) Cost-effectiveness of extending screening mammography guidelines to include women 40–49 years of age, *Annals of Internal Medicine*, 127, 955–65.

Serres, M. (1995) *Michel Serres with Bruno Latour. Conversations on Science, Culture and Time*. Translated by Lapidus, R. Ann Arbor: University of Michigan Press.

Silverman, D. (1993) *Interpreting Qualitative Data. Methods for Analyzing Talk, Text and Interaction.* London: Sage.

Skolbekken, J-A. (1995) The risk epidemic in medical journals, *Social Science and Medicine*, 40, 291–305.

Smith, R. (1991) Rationing: the search for sunlight, *British Medical Journal*, 303, 1561–2.

Spiegelman, D., Colditz, G.A., Hunter, D. *et al.* (1994) Validation of the Gail *et al.* model for predicting individual breast cancer risk, *Journal of the National Cancer Institute*, 86, 600–8.

Stake, R.E. (2000) 'Case Studies'. In Denzin, N.K. and Lincoln, Y.S. (eds) *Handbook of Qualitative Research*. 2nd. Edition. London: Sage.

Tischkowitz, M., Wheeler, D., France, E., Chapman, C., Lucassen, A., Sampson, J., Harper, P., Krawczak, M. and Gray, J. (2000) A comparison of methods currently used in clinical practice to estimate familial breast cancer risks. *Annals of Oncology*, 11, 4, 451–4.

Vasen, H.F.A., Mecklin, J-P., Merakhan, P. and Lynch, H.T. (1991) The international collaborative group on hereditary non-polyposis colorectal cancer. *Diseases of the Colon and Rectum*, 34, 424–5.

Wright, C.J. and Barber Mueller, C. (1995) Screening mammography and public health policy: the need for perspective, *Lancet*, 346, 29–32.

Yin, R.K. (1994) *Case Study Research. Design and Methods.* 2nd. Edition. London: Sage Publications.

3

Governmentality and risk: setting priorities in the new NHS

Paul Joyce

Introduction

The National Health Service (NHS) seeks to provide a comprehensive health care system for the British population. In this chapter it will be argued that the problematisation of health care for which the NHS became the preferred solution, was directly related to a particular discourse of welfare liberal governance that rendered lived reality amenable to political calculation. In essence, the NHS became an institution of collective social insurance with the aim of managing health care resources within the post-war welfare state. However, empirical evidence in the form of interview data will be presented to illustrate how the NHS reforms of the 1980s and 1990s are part of a shift to a neo-liberal formula of governance which articulated a 'free market' rationale as the basis of social policy. Using the conceptual framework of 'governmentality' (associated with the French social theorist Michel Foucault), it will be argued that one of the most important aspects of this shift is that neo-liberal forms of health governance re-code and re-problematise the function of the health care system, predominantly in terms of an economics discourse. The consequence of this new articulation is that the concepts of priority-setting and rationing become embedded as dominant discourses and emergent practices within health policy. This process of re-coding entails reinterpreting the provision of health care services within the NHS as historically a form of *implicit* rationing. The new health economics discourse presents a form of *explicit* rationing as a reasoned and ethical response to the contemporary problem of maximising the benefits of health care within a state-funded and predominantly state-provided health care system.

Since the 1970s, and particularly in the 1980s and 1990s, the question of setting priorities for health care spending has become an increasingly problematic issue within the political regulation of the NHS. The command economy structure of the NHS was increasingly challenged by an economic and political doctrine that questioned the role of the welfare state within society. With the election in 1979 of a radical government that espoused a political doctrine based on neo-liberal economic theory, a search began for new 'market' solutions to problems previously thought not to be amenable to economic discourse. Increasingly the work of the health economist was seen to offer a technical solution to the problem of setting priorities within the NHS and to offer the prospect of 'de-politicising' the whole priorities issue (see Ashmore *et al.* 1989). This would be a 'rational' solution that might result in the health needs of the populations being met more efficiently within a morally justifiable pattern of priorities. Any shift in the health discourse, however, will have a profound effect on other aspects of health governance. It will be argued that a shift to a new health discourse will change the relationship between medical expertise and bureaucratic control and manifest itself in new forms of management structure. Equally important, the shift in the health discourse would alter the relationship between the individual and health care governance. It is argued that it is precisely these types of issues that can be usefully explored using a form of 'governmentality' analysis (see also: Flynn 1997, Hughes and Griffiths 1999, Light 2001).

Governmentality

Foucault defined governmentality as the 'institutions, procedures, analyses and reflections, the calculations and tactics' that support a particular rationale of power and apparatuses of security, with populations as their target (Foucault 1978: in Burchell *et al.* 1991: 102). In effect, governmentality links the techniques of discipline and control of individual living bodies (bio-politics) explored in Foucault's earlier works (such as *The Birth of the Clinic* 1973), directly to state policies. However, unlike more traditional forms of analysis of state power, governmentality shifts the focus of interest from the institutions towards the *practices* of government. These practices are in turn directly related to, and are legitimised by, a 'rationale of government'. Furthermore, the power/knowledge regimes that underpin the rationale of government cannot be identified with the interests of one particular group or groups (see Smart 1986). The fields of power created by a particular power/knowledge discourse simply *exist*. Governmental power and government itself are as much a product of a discourse as the individuals that are subjectified by it. The state becomes a fiction, the central idea of sovereignty part of the rationale of government. Government becomes defined in terms of the 'conduct of conduct', as 'a form of activity aiming to shape, guide or affect the conduct of some person or persons' (Gordon 1991: 2).

The power of governmentality is that it allows the investigation of different aspects of liberal forms of government as essentially different aspects of the problematisation of power (see Rose and Miller 1992, Rose 1993).

The difference between this and traditional policy studies is the notion that conceptions of government and population are not fixed but are the product of the changing power/knowledge discourse in which they are embedded. For Foucault, the Western 'art' of liberal government is a dynamic, self-critical process. At its centre is the inherent tension between minimum intervention by the state and a 'will to knowledge' about populations that expands the number of the categorisations that individuals are subjected to and subjectified by, in the pursuit of the most efficient form of government. However, the reflexive nature of liberalism as a mentality of government, continuously leads to the questioning of appropriate boundaries between the political/public domain of government activity and the non-political/private domain, the preserve of the autonomous individual. The problem for all types of liberalism is that most of the regulation of the population takes place in the non-political/private domain, particularly within the structure of the family. It is in this context that the concept of expertise has evolved as a technology of control and surveillance so that liberal governments can regulate this private domain, 'without destroying its existence and its autonomy' (Rose and Miller 1992: 180).

In this context, the medical profession can be seen as an archetypal form of expertise within liberalism – especially so within welfare liberal forms of governmentality. Indeed, governmentality analysis would suggest that the closer the state becomes associated with the delivery of welfare provision or health care the more well defined and institutionalised professional autonomy becomes. Moreover, as Rose and Miller (1992) suggest, there is a possibility that devolved bureaucratic control combined with the exclusive technical knowledge of expertise will lead to 'enclosures'. In essence a form of reification of the networks of regulatory authority that can be defended and built upon that institutionalise medical expertise and its particular concept of health. Traditionally, within welfare liberalism this 'medical' model of health is essentially curative in nature tending to subjectify the individual as a passive consumer of collective health care provision. However, the relationship between the state, professional expertise and the subjectification of the individual within a power/knowledge discourse is not fixed. When the form of liberal governance changes so will the function of autonomous expertise and its relation to the state within the new 'mentality' of government. As an illustration, within neo-liberalism, collective welfarism is re-coded as a threat to the functioning of the state by virtue of the burden it places on the economy and in the malign way it which it creates a supposed culture of dependency and passivity. This is anathema to the principal dynamic of neo-liberalism that is to be found in the concept of 'the market'. This leads to the assertion that free market economics is

> capable in principle of addressing the totality of human behaviour, and, consequently, of envisaging a coherent, purely economic method of programming the totality of governmental action (Gordon 1991: 43).

The consequences of this are that in the new form of liberal governmentality the state will devise new mechanisms of control and institutions that reflect a different relationship with regulatory expertise and a subtly different subjectification of the individual within the new power/knowledge discourse.

The Conservative governments of the 1980s and 1990s were a prime example of this re-problematisation in action. These administrations instigated a radical programme of reform in part guided by the central tenets of the free market. The privatisation of nationalised industries and utilities, competitive tendering for services and deregulation, can all be seen as part of a reformulation of liberalism in terms of minimal government and 'rolling back the state'. For those sectors of governmental responsibility, such as the NHS, that were previously deemed unsuitable for exposure to the full rigours of the free market, reforms attempted to mimic the mechanisms of the market and create new methodologies to regain control from entrenched professional interest. Thus, the purchaser/provider split and the introduction of the internal market in the NHS were devised to provide the basis of a managed, quasi-market in health care. These were accompanied by the creation of a set of new targets to be met. For example; targets for the reduction of waiting lists, strict guidelines on the return on capital, careful monitoring of the number of patients treated and Finished Consultant Episodes (FCEs), and so on. As Osborne (1997) argues these are consistent with neo-liberal technologies' production of 'surrogate' variables

that will stand measure for otherwise abstract ideas of health . . . Neo-liberalism abandons the quest for an absolute that would be 'health' and opts for determinant strategies, targets and specifics instead (1997: 185).

But this represents more than just the reorganisation of the bureaucratic management of medical expertise; neo-liberal health policy incorporates a new paradigm for health care. As already stated, neo-liberalism is predicated on individuals taking responsibility for their own health and not relying passively on the state. This manifests itself in the emergence of ideas surrounding the concept of a 'new regime of total health care' and a re-emphasis on public health encapsulated in the concept of the 'new public health'.

The construction of the individual in the 'health' discourse

The focus of governmentality analysis is, at its most basic, an investigation of the discursive space that 'renders reality thinkable in such a way that it is amenable to political deliberation' (Rose and Miller 1992: 179). Extending this analysis to health care, one could argue that particular forms of health-needs assessment and the 'new public health' concept are all aspects of a problematisation within a discursive space that makes health care amenable to political action. To be more specific, it is more appropriate to characterise these phenomena as part of a *re*-problematisation of the 'health' discourse, as part of a shift in the articulation of liberal governance from collective forms of welfare to one that emphasises individual rights and responsibilities. The renewed emphasis on public health recognises that,

> many contemporary health problems are... seen as being social rather that solely individual problems; underlying them are concrete issues of local and national public policy, and what are needed to address these problems are 'Healthy Public Policies' – policies in many fields that support the promotion of health (Ashton and Seymour 1988: 21).

In defining health as something more than the absence of illness, agencies charged with the duty to generate 'health' need to make it part of a 'calculus of health' in order to demonstrate effectiveness. An understanding of health in terms of quality of life, as in the 'new public health' formula, is one such approach. The health agency, therefore, has to show that for a given allocation of resources it is trying to maximise the aggregate level of quality of life for its population. One of the consequences of this is that the agency will emphasise preventative strategies as part of health promotion. To maximise aggregate 'health', however, health promotion must focus on individual behaviour (see McQueen 1989).

One characteristic of defining population health as being dependent on individual behaviour is that it becomes part of the duties of the responsible citizen not to indulge in those behaviours likely to result in ill-health and thus add to the burden on society through the extra provision of health care. However, since most of these behaviours are as commonplace as not eating the right food or drinking too much, then the implication is that we are all at risk of adding to aggregate levels of ill-health. The result of this is that the shift away from curative medicine towards health promotion and a new public health agenda in effect becomes a process of privatising health risk. In other words, the collectivisation of welfarism gives way to the privatisation and individualisation of risk which manifests itself in the duty of citizens to act prudently as consumers of health care (see O'Malley 1992). The health agency, therefore, in terms of the 'new public health' discourse, is really in the business of managing health risk. In effect, the management of health risk becomes the most fundamental form of governance with the neo-liberal health discourse. This is, however, a two way process. The individual is expected to perform a kind of self-governance of those aspects of lifestyle which increase the risk of ill health. On the other hand, as illustrated by the example of β-Interferon described later, the agencies of the state through their role as managers of collective risk, have some duty to individuals to provide resources to combat unavoidable risk. It is this tension between the management of collective and individual risk that informs neo-liberal health care governance.

To investigate these issues in greater detail, it is necessary to undertake detailed studies of health service managers' accounts of their practice. The empirical evidence outlined in this section will seek to establish whether the concerns outlined above are reflected in the stated rationales of those charged with the duty of commissioning health care in the NHS – health authorities. It will be argued that the role of *commissioning* given to health authorities as part of the reform process embodies many of the key elements of the new form of health governance. The term commissioning as applied to the post-1991 health authorities implies a strategic understanding of how to meet local health care needs through the appropriate purchasing of health care. As such it is argued that this new role represents a major departure from the traditional role of management within the NHS. Rather than acting as administrators of the health care system they are now required to be pro-active and willing to instigate change to meet these ends.

Selection and analysis of health authorities and community health councils (CHCs)

Empirical evidence is derived from semi-structured interviews (n = 23) conducted separately with the Chief Executives and principal directors of six English health authorities from two NHS regions. The interviews took place between July 1996 and January 1997. Additionally, interviews were conducted between March and July 1997 with a selection of Chief Officers of CHCs (n = 9) that operated in the districts of the sample authorities. The authorities were selected after a review of Purchasing Plan/Commissioning Intentions for 1996/97 from those authorities that outlined a clear priority setting agenda. An additional factor in the selection process was the authority's anticipated future growth potential vis-à-vis the revised funding formula. It was a function of the selection procedure to include as many variables as possible within such a small sample of six authorities. Within the sample there are several different types of authority – city, urban/rural etc., a range of population sizes, variable levels of GP fundholding. Additionally, two of the authorities were committed to locality funding with one discussing it as a future option. In terms of funding, three authorities were below their target allocations and three above target, one significantly so. However, at the time the interviews took place the authorities had not received official notification of their allocations for the financial year 1996/97, and so had to indulge in speculation as to future growth monies. The implications of the funding formula, therefore, had not at that time been fully assimilated and incorporated into future funding plans. As it turned out, 1996/97, being a pre-election year, the allocation for the NHS was a little more generous than anticipated.

The health authority interviewees were asked questions relating to three topic areas: organisational structures and authority activity; input into the decision-making process from locality stakeholders; discussion of the authority's priority setting agenda. The CHC respondents were asked a similar set of questions: organisational structures and activities; relationship with the health authority; priority setting. The interviews were then analysed vertically and horizontally, comparing policy across the selected authorities as well as looking at the differentiation of roles and ideologies within each authority. In this chapter each authority has been designated a letter from A to F and standardised titles have been employed for individual interviewees.

Health authorities: new structures and responsibilities

The 'reform' process instigated by the *Working for Patients* white paper (DoH 1989) officially began in April 1991 with the creation of the 'internal market'. Contracting in the first year was restricted so that a 'steady state' could be maintained until purchasers became more comfortable with their new role within the 'reformed' NHS. Subsequent years saw a relaxation of controls as purchasing authorities developed the new organisational skills needed to operate within the internal market. Many studies have described this changing role of purchasing organisations in the early stages of the reform process (see Appleby *et al.* 1992, Appleby 1994, Freemantle *et al.* 1993, Ranadé 1995). The new role of purchasing was accompanied by changes to the purchasing organisations themselves. Many health authorities merged with their neighbours, leading to a significant reduction in the total number of authorities. In 1991 there were 190 health authorities, by 1994 there were 108. Additionally, health authorities and Family Health Service Authorities (FHSAs) were merged in April 1996 to produce single authorities responsible for the full range of purchasing. At the same time as the average size of health authorities was increasing, the level of GP fund-holding was also increasing and becoming an important factor in overall purchasing activity. By 1994 the proportion of the population covered by fundholding was 36 per cent, by 1996 it had risen to around half the population (Audit Commission 1996, Ranadé 1997). Another significant change was the level of services provided by organisations with Trust status. The initial wave of Trust applications accounted for approximately 13 per cent of NHS expenditure. This had risen to 95 per cent by the fourth wave in 1994 (Smee 1995).

By 1996, when the initial interviews took place, the level of merger activity had declined from its peak in 1991–94. Each authority in the sample had already merged with their FHSAs. There were no Directly Managed Units (DMU) providing health care in the district. Contracting arrangements had been in place for several years and GP fundholding was an established practice in all districts. Moreover, the purchasing role was beginning to move out of the shadow of the supply-side provider interests that had dominated the thinking of policy makers when the internal market was created (see Ham 1994). The initial reform process, as Hunter states:

> was almost exclusively concerned with introducing supply-side changes without really attending to the question of what the changes were actually for (Hunter 1993: 33).

Therefore, because of its original inchoate nature it becomes doubly important to examine how the role of purchasing and commissioning has developed within the 'reformed' NHS.

Organisational structures: commissioning local health care services

In an earlier study of eight purchasing authorities, Freemantle *et al.* (1993) distinguished between two distinct organisational structures; one dominated by directorate function (finance, public health, planning etc.); the other having a flatter managerial structure with more cross-directorate input into the decision-making process. To some extent the evidence from the current sample of six authorities on the whole supports this analysis. All of the six authorities in the survey described their current managerial structures in terms of having moved, or as in the process of moving, away from a rigid directorate structure to the cross-directorate or 'mixed matrix' model. The declared rationale behind this transition was the clear desire to deliver a 'change agenda' that focused on the broader concept of 'commissioning' instead of the 'technical' exercises of purchasing and contracting. Moreover, each of the authorities perceived the primary role of commissioning to be the development of a strategic overview in order to meet health needs in the district through the operation of effective and appropriate purchasing and contracting.

The notion that commissioning is qualitatively different from the technical function of purchasing or contracting was reflected in the interview data with all health authority directors. The comments of the Director of Public Health below are typical of a 'holistic' understanding of commissioning expressed by respondents:

> Commissioning is strategic overview, but also much more involvement with other agencies. Whereas contracting tends to be only those we are actually giving money to. If I could put it as crudely as that (Director of Public Health, HA C).

As the above illustrates, the 'strategic' nature of commissioning implies forging new relationships with other agencies, with the medical profession and with local people whose health needs are to be met. It was clear from the interviews, however, that even though all were actively engaged in changing their management structures to operationalise their new strategic function, health authorities were still evolving a language of strategic planning that could conceptualise this new role in a coherent way.

Rationing, priority-setting and health needs assessment

The shift in rhetoric to include the ideas of meeting health needs and of 'health gain' effectively opened up the concept of health to include the potential for pro-active interventions by strategic management. The use of health promotion and disease prevention strategies, focusing on 'risky' behaviour indulged in by individuals, clearly resembles the 'new public health' concept mention earlier. As one Director of Commissioning argued:

> The strategic framework, and a lot of the work that supports that, is about trying to change the language and change the approach... You are actually using different language about health gain, for instance, which is important language. But then, within that we are talking about personal responsibility for your own health. How do you involve local populations in that debate? How do you make people aware of their responsibilities? What responsibilities do they have to the health service in their use of the health service? Then you are moving on to their opinions about priorities because you are obviously not going to be able to do everything, which is the rationing debate (Director of Commissioning, HA E).

As the above example suggests, one of the consequences of making health care choices, either individually or collectively, is that the vexed question of priority-setting inevitably raises its head. One of the criteria for selecting the authorities in the research sample was the inclusion of a set of well defined priority goals in their purchasing plans or commissioning intentions. Many of the sample authorities ranked these goals in terms of high, medium or low priorities. Only one authority, however, included in their purchasing plan a detailed list of services that the authority had decided *not* to purchase as extra contractual referrals (ECRs) – except in circumstances of 'overriding clinical need'. The document was very explicit in its description of the services to be excluded. In character, it closely resembled the type of selection criteria produced by Berkshire HA that had made front page national news some months earlier (Crail 1995).

Simply reading purchasing plans might lead any researcher to the easy conclusion that this authority, together with a handful of others, was alone in having a strict rationing policy. However, it was clear from discussions with other authorities in the sample that this was far from a unique occurrence. All the other authorities, whether they acknowledged that a formal discussion of exclusions had taken place in the authority or not, had a very similar list of services that they would not purchase except in extreme circumstances. As one Chief Executive described it:

> The classic example – there is nothing new here – tattoos acquired in adult life. But there were others, other areas. Unless there were very significant clinical reasons, breast enlargement... Then orthodontics... Where do we go next? In Vitro, it's slightly more judgmental. But we do have some, 'so far and no further'. You know, we won't go on trying forever... (Chief Executive, HA F).

In practice, the authorities had roughly the same policy with only slight variations in the lists of restricted services. Collating all the lists would produce the same selection of services that have been documented elsewhere (see Redmayne et al. 1993, Redmayne 1995, Klein et al. 1996). However, it can be argued that in reality the restriction criteria amounted to an Extra Contractual Referral (ECR) policy rather than a general policy of explicit rationing.

The more important question that arises from the use of these rationing/ECR policies is whether they could form a template for future activity that will lead to a more generalised debate on priorities. The response from the authorities pointed to something of a dilemma. The production of the restricted lists was seen as relatively straightforward, formalising restriction that already existed on authority activity. However, when questioned about whether the selection criteria used in the creation of restricted lists would ultimately change historical patterns of core services the replies were more guarded, as the comments of a Director of Finance testify:

> It ought to. The question is whether we are there or not. Whether we can actually support that from a public health viewpoint, from a health needs viewpoint and a clinical effectiveness viewpoint. Big debate there (Director of Finance, HA E).

It was evident from similar replies that none of the sample authorities had yet engaged in that 'big debate' about priorities. This reluctance, however, was not the result of a lack of sophistication in their approach to health care. It pointed more to an instinctive pragmatism when faced with the limitations of relying on supposedly more rational ways of doing things. It was clear that all the authorities in the sample were well aware of the new possibilities that the reform process had given them to influence the health agenda. Each authority felt that that they had many more instruments to make change than they had previously and were on the whole optimistic about making real and substantial changes to the mix of services in the long run. It is equally fair to say, however, that the authorities in the survey still felt that making any substantial changes was proving to be difficult and only really possible at the margins of activity. Moreover, they asserted that many of the obstacles in the way of making strategic choices were the product of perverse incentives built into the system that prevented them from fulfilling their remit to the fullest extent. Furthermore, these obstructions were not financial or managerial but political.

Political regulation of the Health Service

It would be wrong to suggest that all forms of political macro-level regulation were seen by the authorities as antagonistic to their strategic commissioning role. Many of the key strategic targets set by the political centre, such as the *Health of the Nation* initiatives or a 'primary health care led' NHS, were entirely consistent with the wider understanding of health and health care that looks at quality of life rather than absence of disease. Moreover, many of these initiatives reflect quintessentially 'new public health' ideas of personal responsibility and the self-management of health risk. All the authorities felt comfortable that they could accommodate most of these targets within their overall commissioning strategy – with a little modification to suit local circumstances. However, what perplexed many respondents was the feeling that the total number of directives from the centre (and regionally) left them little room to manoeuvre, and many times contradicted their responsibility to act strategically to meet perceived local needs. Interestingly, the most pessimistic were the Directors of Public Health. The response of one Director of Public Health when asked about the degree to which the authority was constrained by national priorities illustrates the point. As she stated:

> At the moment totally. The first national priority is not to give us any extra money. But having said that we were talking the other day about Health of the Nation, with cancer Calmanisation, with pressure on intensive care beds, with pressures on medical emergency admissions, with pressure on us improving our access to renal services. They are all priorities raining down. I feel like there is no room at all (Director of Public Health, HA C).

What concerned all the authorities, however, was the political imperative from the centre to increase activity that could demonstrate the 'success' of the government's day-to-day stewardship of the health system. Especially problematic was the measure of activity encapsulated in the 'efficiency index'. The efficiency index seeks to measure activity within the NHS by monitoring the number of Finished Consultant Episodes or FCEs generated by a health care episode. In essence the efficiency index is a proxy measure of 'value for money' but does so using a very narrow criterion biased in favour of acute activity. Every health authority was given an index target to meet and so had to ensure that Trusts, who actually provided the measured activity, also met their targets. Without exception, the efficiency index was the topic that elicited the strongest comments from respondents. The comments of a Director of Public Health illustrate this point:

> I mean FCEs. The biggest way to flannel figures is to look at FCEs.
> I mean again, if I went into hospital and I was seen by six different consultants, that's six different FCEs. I'm only the one body lying in the one bed and I might have seen the six of them during a two-day period. And then we get these wondrous statements that the NHS is seeing more patients than ever. Baloney! Or words to that effect (Director of Public Health, HA D).

For most authorities in the sample, simply meeting the efficiency index target was not seen as an issue. The more problematic area was that many authorities wanted to reduce acute activity, as their commissioning intentions had indicated, but they could not do so without having to manipulate the efficiency figures. This meant maximising efficiency gains from acute Trusts to compensate for increases in activity elsewhere. The general impression was that the authorities treated the efficiency index with some disdain fundamentally because it distracted the authority from their 'proper' role of commissioning.

The general feeling was that efficiency indexes, like waiting lists, were part of the political 'game' which had to be entered into by authorities whether they thought it relevant or not. When it comes to comparing micro (providers), meso (strategic purchasers) and macro (political) influence over the reformed health system, it is clear from the last series of comments that purchasing authorities felt constrained by macro-level priorities. What was unclear, however, was the degree to which this political dimension was in turn influenced by 'the ability of interest groups ... to manipulate public opinion to their advantage' (Freemantle *et al.* 1993: 547). This is indeed an important point which will be explored in the next section. However, the main finding that stems from the analysis of this macro level of governance is not that formal political control is problematic because it is susceptible to external influence but because it uses an intrinsic calculus of regulatory control that is often antagonistic to other levels of governance.

User/carer groups

One important set of interest groups that has yet to be mentioned in the context of commissioning health care are the numerous user/carer organisations. All the authorities in the sample emphasised their sensitivity to the opinion of users and carers when developing new services, reorganising existing ones or restricting access to marginal treatments. The comments below by a Director of Public Health were typical of the responses from directors.

> I think the other major way of consulting with people is though the service reviews and making sure that the local voluntary groups, the users groups, the carers groups are involved because it is much more real when you are talking about the needs of people with disabilities, or whatever, there is something crisp to catch hold on rather than nebulous global health issues (Director of Public Health, HA C).

For authorities, the obvious advantage of working with such groups was that they directly represented consumer/patient interests and needs or were the consumers themselves. However, caution was also expressed that many of the groups were by nature partisan, and this needed to be taken into consideration when including them in service development discussions. Another problem with these groups, it was suggested, was that difficulties would arise when there existed different factions within the same area of concern – all competing for attention.

The key body within each health authority charged with the responsibility of representing local interests is the Community Health Council, a concession to the early 1970s conception of consumerism. However, it was clear from the interview data that many (five out of six health authorities and a majority of the CHC directors interviewed) thought that the CHCs were marginal to authority activities. Especially in the production of the annual Purchasing Plan and general strategic thinking, CHCs were 'recipients rather than shapers and influencers'. As one Chief Officer stated when asked about the CHC's influence on changing health authority priorities,

> If the health authority was a thousand miles long, about half an inch. [laughs] Not a lot... one gets the impression time and time again that they have already decided what they are going to do and the CHC gets invited to sort of twiddle around the edges' (Chief Officer, CHC C).

Even some of those authorities that attested to good working relations with CHCs attributed this to the fact that 'they don't cause us a problem'. On the whole, there seemed to be little enthusiasm from health authorities to include CHCs in their discussions. The CHC was 'still a distant, kept-at-arms length, organisation' (Health Authority Director) (see Appleby *et al.* 1992, Dunham and Smith 1993).

However, it was clear from the interview data that user/carer groups had other ways of directly influencing the priority-setting debate. One of the examples most often cited by health authority directors of user/carer influence was in the introduction of new, and many times unproven, drug therapies. One such therapy that was a concern to all authorities was that of β-Interferon for the treatment of Multiple Sclerosis. The debate about the introduction of these new and usually very expensive drug therapies has been documented elsewhere (for example Freemantle and Harrison 1993, on Interleukin-2). The case of β-Interferon is just one of a number of new high profile drug treatments that have been developed by drug companies either as a means of treating previously intractable conditions or as safer and more effective treatments than established drug regimes. The controversy surrounding these drug treatments highlights a number of problems for health authorities seeking to retain control of their own priority setting agenda in the light of political pressure from the centre. This is made even more difficult when there is a difference of opinion between medical professionals and user/carer groups over the efficacy of such treatments.

The case of β-Interferon

The case of β-Interferon illustrates some of the difficulties faced by health authorities in coping with new drugs designed to treat diseases for which previously there were no effective drug treatments. Moreover, the case of β-Interferon highlights how different levels of governance – micro (providers), meso (strategic purchasers) and macro (political) – and the interests of different groups interact when difficult priority decisions have to be made. β-Interferon is the first new product to treat (but not cure) the chronic disease of Multiple Sclerosis (MS), especially for patients with the relapse-remitting form of the disease and without significant disability. The drug has the effect of reducing the frequency of relapses as the disease process progresses. For this reason β-Interferon has been described as a 'drug company's dream-ticket', in that MS is incurable, relatively common and that β-Interferon is fairly expensive (Rous *et al.* 1996: 1195). The cost works out at approximately £10,000 per patient per year or £33,000 per relapse avoided (Richards 1996: 1159). It has been estimated that if all the patients in the UK with relapse-remitting MS (45 per cent of the total) were to be treated with β-Interferon then the total cost might be as much as £380m per annum – equivalent to 10 per cent of the total drugs bill (see New 1996).

Clearly, uncontrolled prescribing of β-Interferon would have had a major impact on health authority spending. In recognition of this a guidance letter was produced by the NHS Executive on prescribing the drug (NHSE EL (95)97). The drug would only be available through consultants at regional centres and each authority – in collaboration with the MS Society – would have to devise a protocol for its use that would set in place patient selection criteria. However, what worried the authorities in the sample was not the problems associated with protocol production but that β-Interferon had set a precedent for the introduction of *other* contentious drug therapies. The most problematic aspect was the absence of debate about the impact these drugs would have on the allocation of resources to meet other more pressing local priorities. This concern is illustrated by the response from a Director of Public Health.

> Take drugs. There are two decisions. One is in principle, is this a drug that the NHS should be providing? The second decision is, if it should be provided, for whom and under what circumstances? The first of those decisions on β-Interferon was taken by default – 'β-Interferon is a good thing' – from on high. The problem then was managing the introduction and that was about protocols and so on, and health authorities putting aside development money if they could. That process is starting to be used as a template for other drugs and other technologies. I'm a little concerned about that, because if I am straightaway into a debate about how do I manage the introduction of things, and for whom should it be available, it begs the question of whether it should be in the first place, and I don't think there is yet a mechanism for asking those questions, that initial question (Director of Public Health, HA B).

This concern was echoed in other authorities. As Rous *et al.* point out:

> Purchasers were unable to decline funding for a marginally effective drug and thereby undertake explicit rationing. To ensure prescribing was within the guidelines, a vast communication network had to be sustained with managers, general practitioners, neurologists, the Multiple Sclerosis Society, and professional advisers in all the purchasing authorities. The workload involved was considerable (Rous *et al.* 1996: 1196).

However, the lack of debate about purchasing at authority level did not prevent a lively debate within the medical profession from developing. The medical evidence about β-Interferon and its long-term effectiveness was disputed by several senior neurologists. It was suggested that β-Interferon should not be made widely available and that resources would be better spent on other kinds of support for MS sufferers (McDonald 1995, also see Drug Therapeutics 1996). It was apparent that some of those who opposed the introduction of β-Interferon felt that the proper evaluation procedures had not been adhered to and that non-clinical values had prevailed.

In response to such claims the chief executive of the MS Society emphasised the 'responsible way the MS Society [had] sought to work with those managing this complex situation' (Cardy 1997: 600). Furthermore, he stated:

> The MS Society has worked hard to ensure access to authoritative information and to reduce expectations. As a result, patients in Britain have not made a stampede for interferon beta (1997: 600).

On the whole, the experience of sample authorities reinforced this sentiment and expressed satisfaction with the production of the protocol. There were no reported serious problems with the MS Society and, in general, it was stated that they had acted 'responsibly' in the protocol discussions. One director, however, suggested that they had unrealistic expectations of the effectiveness of the drug, and that the MS Society thought β-Interferon was 'the best thing since sliced bread'.

At the core of the controversy over the introduction of β-Interferon is the question of effectiveness. It was clear that one of the key elements in the dispute between representatives of MS sufferers and the medical profession about the usefulness of the drug was to do with the different values each group attached to patients' state of health. For some neurologists, the important factor in opposing the introduction of β-Interferon was that it '[had] no significant effect on the development of disease in multiple sclerosis' (Harvey 1996: 297). The narrowness of this view based on clinical indicators and ultimate end-states for patients was starkly at odds with the views of many patients where the reduction in frequency in relapse was seen to be a justifiable goal in itself (see Burnfield 1997). It is apparent that many MS sufferers view β-Interferon as a legitimate use of resources to meet an unavoidable health risk. The potential improvement in the quality-of-life for sufferers is itself justification enough. However, in terms of clinical measures of post-treatment outcomes based on changes in the physical health status of the patient, these quality of life values were not readily amenable to calculation as part of a general disability measure. It is therefore apparent that when there are conflicting but equally valid ways of conceptualising outcomes, the measurement of effectiveness will be compromised. And if effectiveness is the criterion that informs the priority-setting debate then the transparency and explicitness of the debate will also be compromised.

The clear implication of β-Interferon is that the views of user/carer groups cannot be directly incorporated into health authority commissioning plans. The disparate and partisan nature of the groups will often result in conflict with the strategic aims of commissioning. Health authorities are compelled by their commissioning remit to allocate resources to meet the health needs of the local population as a whole. The demands of particular groups for more resources have to be balanced against the equally legitimate claims of other groups and the needs of the local population. However, the example of β-Interferon illustrates that this balancing act may prove problematic for commissioning health authorities. The lack of an explicit debate about priorities indicates that there is no language of prioritisation in which competing claims for resources can be discussed rationally and without emotion. Moreover, the use of governmentality analysis strongly indicates that the failure of such a language to evolve appears to be a function of that particular form of governance rather that a lack of will on the part of health care commissioners.

Concluding comments

The evidence previously outlined leads to the conclusion that the development of the strategic purchasing role within health authorities has produced a very consistent set of management structures that reflect a common understanding of the commissioning remit. Despite some minor differences of emphasis, the interview data suggest that all the purchasing authorities saw it as their duty to make real changes in service provision to meet local health needs. However, despite this expression of commitment to their commissioning remit, all the authorities in the sample felt that they were hampered to some degree by the priorities imposed from the centre. This reinforces the observation that micro, meso and macro levels of governance often work against each other even though they are all products of the same neo-liberal form of health governance. This in itself provides a valuable critique of totalising and deterministic discourses of governance. The fracturing of health governance has major implications for health policy. It is evident that the tension between the macro, meso and micro levels of governance is an inherent part of this form of neo-liberal governance of health care. Therefore, the fact that each 'level' of governance has different, and often conflicting, criteria with which to judge success or failure implies that the de-politicisation of administration is unachievable.

As the evidence presented suggests, this conflict within governance has meant that purchasing authorities lacked the means or vocabulary to embark on a full-scale priorities debate. It has to be emphasised, however, that this was not because of any lack of enthusiasm. All the authorities had embarked on a limited process of formulating local priorities, but this was mostly at the margins of authority activity (*i.e.* ECRs), which had little impact on overall priority arrangements. The question posed was whether these small-scale attempts to bring some kind of 'rationality' to the priorities debate could be scaled-up to become the basis of a 'big debate' on priorities. This research shows that this did not seem to be happening and probably will not happen. On the one hand, authorities seemed to be daunted by the enormity and complexity of devising global strategies. The response was to fall back onto a form of pragmatic incrementalism, aided by the use of managerial technologies such as audit and effectiveness criteria. On the other hand, authorities, in their guise as commissioners of health care services, lacked a conceptual language of priority-setting to legitimate essentially moral decisions about priorities. The absence of a unifying priorities discourse is made more apparent when authorities incorporated other groups, such as user/care representatives, into the strategic commissioning process. The case of β-Interferon illustrates this point. The evidence suggested that these groups were useful to authorities because they were able to bring an un-mediated understanding of user and carer health needs to commissioning. However, user/carer involvement in commissioning was treated with suspicion by some directors because of the fragmented and partisan nature of the groups. Even so, it was evident that a number of the sample authorities considered user/carer groups to have more influence over the commissioning process than the official consumer representatives in the district, the Community Health Councils.

Again, using a governmentality approach, the substantive point is that this fracturing of the consumer voice into several potentially conflicting agendas is not to be viewed as a 'failure' of health governance to be rectified, but is an intrinsic part of it. Moreover, the means by which this neo-liberal economic discourse is re-conceptualised within health governance (so as to make health amenable to a new form of political/economic calculation) can only be achieved by a concomitant re-conceptualisation of consumer sovereignty. In effect, the commissioning authorities have to construct a proxy consumer in the form of an aggregation of a disparate collection of personal risks, local needs and individual desires. It is arguably the case, however, that many groups will legitimately represent consumer values even if they do conflict with others (as in the case of β-Interferon). Therefore, the totality of consumer opinion cannot be accessed through these groups. For specific developments this is often acceptable, but in terms of the 'big priorities debate' it falls well short of what is needed.

One of the strengths of governmentality analysis is that it can be still applied even though new political regimes come to power with ostensibly different ideologies of government. The election in 1997 of a new Labour government illustrates this point. The new regime's first substantive document on the future direction for the NHS, the White Paper entitled *The New NHS: Modern, Dependable* (DoH 1997: 11) appears to offer a new vision for the health service. The new government committed itself to the abolition of the internal market (but retaining the 'purchaser/provider split') and to replace contracts with long-term 'service level agreements'. However, the main change is in the commissioning function. The plan as outlined in the White Paper, is that the primary responsibility for purchasing and 'commissioning' will be gradually devolved, over a four-stage process, to 'primary care groups' dominated by medical professionals.

In effect, the proposals in the White Paper restrict the District Health Authority's role to that of the former Regional Health Authorities. However, the detail of the new health authority role is not really the issue under discussion. The more important question is whether the new plans for the NHS represent a shift in the formula of health governance? In other spheres of government activity – social security, education and law and order – many of the themes associated with neo-liberal governance such as personal responsibility and questioning the limits of government activity, are being articulated as part of new Labour philosophy. The new arrangements for health authorities raise a number of key issues discussed earlier, such as management control over the priority decisions and forms of legitimacy. Indeed, many of the problems are heightened by the proposed changes, especially the problem of maintaining strategic oversight and overcoming the traditional individualistic culture of medical professionals. Moreover, many of the key technologies associated with the previous form of management, such as audit- and evidence-based medicine, will be retained. In fact their use will be institutionalised through the creation of the 'National Institute for Clinical Effectiveness' (NICE) and the 'Commission for Health Improvement' (CHI), to disseminate good practice (for treatments such as β-Interferon) and monitor quality standards. Clearly, the most radical difference is in the creation of the 'primary care groups' to take over commissioning, which, ironically, have echoes of Enthoven's original plan for the NHS (modelled on the Health Maintenance Organisation (HMO) system in the US) that was the source of so much controversy for the previous Conservative regime.

Using the Foucauldian framework of 'governmentality' it can be seen that the discourse of commissioning, rationing and priority-setting in the NHS, and the institutional practices in which it is embedded, operate at a much more fundamental level than surface political activity would indicate. It is clear that the shift to a neo-liberal form of governance (and the subsequent shift to a neo-liberal form of health governance) has created a new means of conceptualising lived reality – a process of making it amenable to political calculation. This new mentality of liberal government creates a discursive space in which political activity becomes 'thinkable' and which in turn defines the ambitions and limits of policy action. Therefore, it is clear that radical change in the governance of health care only comes about through a shift in the problematisation of liberal governance, not merely in the transition from one political regime to another.

References

Appleby, J. (1994) *Developing Contracting: a National Survey of District Health Authorities, Boards and NHS Trusts*. Research Paper 15. Birmingham: NAHAT.

Appleby, J., Little, V., Ranadé, W., Robinson R. and Smith P. (1992) *Implementing the Reforms: a Second National Survey of District General Managers*. Project Paper 7. Birmingham: NAHAT.

Ashmore, M., Mulkay, M. and Pinch, T. (1989) *Health and Efficiency: a Sociology of Health Economics*. Buckingham: Open University Press.

Ashton, J. and Seymour, H. (1988) *The New Public Health*. Milton Keynes: Open University Press.

Audit Commission (1996) *Funding Facts*. London: HMSO.

Burchell, G., Gordon, C. and Miller, P. (eds) (1991) *The Foucault Effect: Studies in Governmentality*. Hemel Hempstead: Harvester Wheatsheaf.

Burnfield, A (1997) Reducing frequency and severity of relapses will be of great clinical benefit, *British Medical Journal*, 314, 600.

Cardy, P. (1997) Relapses deserve treatment, *British Medical Journal*, 314, 600.

Crail, M. (1995) Rational judgements, *Health Service Journal*, 105, 12.

Department of Health (1997) *The New NHS: Modern, Dependable*, London: HMSO.

Department of Health (1989) *Working for Patients*, Cmnd. 855. London: HMSO.

Drug Therapeutics Bulletin (1996) *Interferon Beta 1b – Hope or Hype?*, 34, 9–11.

Dunham, P. and Smith, S. (1993) The changing role of the CHCs, *Health Service Management*, May, 14–16.

Flynn, R. (1997) *'Governmentality' and determinacy in quasi market contracting.* Paper presented at British Sociological Annual Conference, York, 7–10 April.

Foucault, M. (1973) *The Birth of the Clinic: an Archaeology of Medical Perception.* New York: Pantheon Books.

Freemantle, N. and Harrison, S. (1993) Interleukin-2: the public and professional face of rationing in the NHS, *Critical Social Policy*, 13, 3, 94–117.

Freemantle, N., Watt, I. and Mason, J. (1993) Developments in the purchasing process in the NHS: towards an explicit politics of rationing?, *Public Administration*, 71, 535–48.

Gordon, C. (1991) Government rationality: an introduction. In Burchell, G., Gordon, C. and Miller, P. (eds) *The Foucault Effect: Studies in Governmentality.* Hemel Hempstead: Harvester Wheatsheaf.

Ham, C. (1994) *Management and Competition in the New NHS.* Oxford: Radcliffe Medical Press.

Harvey, P. (1996) Why interferon beta 1b was licensed is a mystery, *British Medical Journal*, 313, 297.

Hughes, D. and Griffiths, L. (1999) On penalties and the Patient's Charter: centralism v decentralised governance in the NHS, *Sociology of Health and Illness*, 21, 1, 71–94.

Hunter, D. (1993) *Rationing Dilemmas in Healthcare.* Birmingham: NAHAT.

Klein, R., Day, P. and Redmayne, S. (1996) *Managing Scarcity: Priority Setting and Rationing in the NHS.* Buckingham: Open University Press.

Light, D.W. (2001) Comparative institutional response to economic policy managed competition and governmentality, *Social Science and Medicine*, 52, 8, 1151–66.

McDonald, W.I. (1995) New treatments for multiple sclerosis, *British Medical Journal*, 310, 345–6.

McQueen, D. (1989) Thoughts on the ideological origins of Health Promotion, *Health Promotion*, 4, 4, 339–42.

New, B. (1996) The rationing agenda in the NHS, *British Medical Journal*, 312, 1593–601.

NHS Executive (1995) *New Drugs for Multiple Sclerosis EL(95)97.* Leeds: Department of Health.

O'Malley, P. (1992) Risk, power and crime prevention, *Economy and Society*, 21, 3, 252–75.

Osborne, T. (1997) Of health and statecraft. In Petersen, A. and Bunton, R. (eds) *Foucault, Health and Medicine.* London: Routledge.

Paton, C. (1996) *Health Policy and Management: the Health-care Agenda in a British Political Context.* London: Chapman and Hall.

Ranadé, W. (1995) The theory and practice of managed competition in the National Health Service, *Public Administration*, 73, 241–62.

Redmayne, S. (1995) *Reshaping the NHS: Strategies, Priorities and Resource Allocation*, Research Paper No. 16. Birmingham: NAHAT.

Redmayne, S., Klein, R. and Day, P. (1993) *Sharing Out Resources: Purchasing and Priority Setting in the NHS*, Research Paper No. 11. Birmingham: NAHAT.

Richards, R. G. (1996) Interferon beta in multiple sclerosis: Clinical cost effectiveness falls at the first hurdle, *British Medical Journal*, 313, 1159.

Rose, N. (1993) Government, authority and expertise in advanced liberalism, *Economy and Society*, 22, 3.

Rose, N. and Miller, P. (1992) Political power beyond the state: problematics of government, *British Journal of Sociology*, 43, 2, 173–205.

Rous, E., Coppel, A., Hayworth, J. and Noyce, S. (1996) A purchaser experience of managing new expensive drugs: interferon beta, *British Medical Journal*, 313, 1195–6.

Smart, B. (1986) The politics of truth and the problem of hegemony. In Hoy, D. C. (ed) *Foucault: a Critical Reader*. Oxford: Blackwell.

Smee, C. (1995) Self-governing trusts and GP fundholders: the British experience. In Saltman, R. and Von Otter, C. (eds) *Implementing Planned Markets in Health Care*. Buckingham: Open University Press.

4

Categorisation and micro-rationing: access to care in a French emergency department

Carine Vassy

Introduction

There is a considerable health sociology literature on patient categorisation by health care personnel. It has been shown that staff, acting collectively, construct typical patient profiles and subsequently evaluate presenting persons according to certain expected categories. But, while there are many accounts of categorisation in action, the rationing of care at the micro-level has been neglected. With a few exceptions (Griffiths and Hughes 1994, Timmermans 1999), sociologists have not linked the two concepts. This is partly because interest in micro-level rationing is relatively new, and partly because health sociologists have paid insufficient attention to the practical consequences of categorisation for patient care outcomes. A re-reading of the patient categorisation literature shows that many patients subjected to negative judgements and pejorative labelling also experienced delays in treatment or denial of access to care (two of the basic forms of health care rationing). Patient categorisation leads first, to the formulation of a particular definition of the case, and second, to socially discriminative practices towards the presenting patient concerned. Both the quantity and quality of care given to such patients may be diminished.

If one accepts this linkage between categorisation and rationing, it follows that the latter can be based on many of the factors documented in the categorisation literature. Rationing may depend on perceptions of the condition for which treatment is sought. Thus it has been argued that some conditions are considered as less worthy of care than others, for instance terminal conditions (Glaser and Strauss 1965), psychiatric disorders (Jeffery 1979, Roth 1972) and strokes (Hoffmann 1974). By contrast, other clinical features such as those which constitute the 'interesting case' relevant to medical training, 'mobilise' staff action so that patients gain quicker and more extensive care (Dodier and Camus 1998, Jeffery 1979, Sudnow 1967).

Rationing can also rest on judgements about personal or social character. Patients with similar physical conditions, but with perceived differences of other kinds, may experience differential access to care. Often this will affect individuals who are seen as having low social worth. It has been reported that older people receive fewer resuscitative attempts than younger patients with similar conditions (Sudnow 1967, 1973, Timmermans 1999). Studies also show that persons whose way of life, personal history or putative social class are morally disvalued, like tramps, 'drunks', and drug addicts (Jeffery 1979, Mannon 1976, Roth 1972, Sudnow 1967) are given less, or less good, care. The financial status of the patient, his/her type of employment, his/her insurance protection, or his/her use of private-practice doctors are also stressed by Roth (1972) as factors which affect the quality of care given. Evaluations of patient behaviour in the immediate face-to-face situation can also result in delay or denial of care. Patients who were perceived as unco-operative or over-complaining received less attention in the surgical unit studied by Lorber (1975) and in the psychiatric ward studied by May and Kelly (1982).

As shown in these examples, we should be alert to the possibility that rationing may take a variety of forms, including delay in offering care, a lower ranking in a queue for treatment, less time with hospital staff, the direction of the patient to other less desirable treatment facilities and the direct denial of treatment. The aim of this chapter is to explore the implementation of these last two, most clear-cut forms of rationing in a French emergency department (ED). In the hospital as well as in other human service settings, staff tend to modify the intake processes through which clients enter organisations (Hughes 1971). Staff members act as gatekeepers who control what they see as inappropriate demands for services. They decide whether the incoming person can access the services or not and, if so, his or her rank of priority. EDs are a particularly interesting place for those who want to observe health rationing in action. They are organisations that can be accessed by patients drawn from the entire population, and which lack any single agreed definition about what constitutes an emergency case (Wolcott 1979). The constant increase in ED attendances, particularly in France (circa plus five per cent per year), brings ED staff into contact with greater numbers of presenting patients whose conditions are seen as inappropriate for emergency treatment.

Roth (1972) and Roth and Douglas (1983), in a study of five North American EDs, provide many examples where patients were turned away without treatment. Staff made judgements about the social worth of patients, taking into account such attributes as age, race, sex, behaviour, mode of dress, language and accent. Persons of lower status were more likely to be turned away than others. In the three British EDs studied by Jeffery (1979), staff did not refuse to treat patients but sometimes varied the quality and quantity of care (waiting time, comprehensiveness of the clinical examination, hostile attitudes) according to the perceived characteristics of the case.

Those seen as tramps, 'drunks', drug users, or persons having 'self-inflicted' conditions were negatively evaluated. In another British ED studied by Hughes (1989) few patients were refused access, but one category sometimes turned away were 'regulars' returning to seek further treatment for 'old' injuries after an initial visit a few days earlier. Dodier and Camus (1998) provide another perspective on these issues, based on their study of a French ED. They take issue with the view that the imputation of low social status leads automatically to a reduction in the quality or quantity of a patient's care. The patients thus labelled aroused complex reactions, which ranged from highly negative attitudes to a real 'mobilisation' of resources in their favour. Treatment of these cases was dependent on circumstances (particular flow of patients at the time), and on individual staff attitudes. This study raises the important question of whether past studies over-simplify the picture when they suggest that lower social class attenders are the group most likely to be denied access to care.

Previous ED studies leave many questions unanswered. First, it is unclear what precise roles staff from different occupational groups (doctors, nurses and clerks) play in patient categorisation and how their actions are co-ordinated. One hypothesis is that doctors play a crucial role in framing the rules of patient eligibility, but delegate the implementation of these rules to nurses and reception staff. Hughes (1989) raises the question of the margin of discretion of the gatekeeper, another issue requiring further research. His work suggests that lower-ranking staff (such as clerks) commonly accept the overturning of their decisions by higher-ranking staff (such as doctors) without demur, but it is not clear if this is a general phenomenon. Another question is whether patients can influence the judgement given on them. As was noticed by Kelly and May (1982), categorisation is often analysed with a structural and static approach; not with an interactionist one. It is generally considered that the categorisation criteria are fixed before the patient arrives on the scene, and that the label s/he is given is not negotiable. But it is not certain whether patients, more generally, accept such a passive role in their evaluation. Finally, we still need to know more about how staff weigh the various factors that may contribute to decisions: what happens when there is a contradiction between different criteria, and whether one criterion has overwhelming determinative power?

Generally speaking, sociological studies pay little attention either to specific, local features of EDs, such as unique organisational characteristics of a hospital, or the wider social and political context. A study such as this one, in which all categories of staff were systematically interviewed, allows for a more detailed investigation of the moral principles used in categorising and prioritising patients. It then becomes possible to consider whether there is a consensus about these principles. The supplementation of the interviews with field observations made it possible to examine the 'rules' in action, including the way they were communicated and elaborated through staff members' accounting practices. The analysis that follows pays particular attention to staff notions of ethical work practice and their solidification into what might be called models of 'local justice', as developed by Elster and Herpin (1992). Even though the allocation mechanisms described by these authors (in the field of organ transplants) are more formal and codified than categorisation in the ED, there are many similar features.

The concept of the decision-making process in an organisational context (Crozier 1963, Crozier and Friedberg 1977) has been adopted as an appropriate theoretical framework for understanding the intake process in the ED (see Vassy 1999, for another application of the approach). The 'strategic analysis of organisations' indicates that such decision-making processes depend on a set of informal rules, and associated norms and values. The characteristics of these rules depend on power relationships within the organisation.

Methods and data sources

The data presented in the chapter were gathered in the ED of an 850-bedded French general hospital, which provided general, acute, obstetric and geriatric services. Activity levels in the medical and surgical units of the hospital, including the ED, were increasing. But, because costs exceed revenue, the hospital budget was in deficit. The hospital is located in a deprived Parisian suburb. There is a large immigrant population and the unemployment rate is high. The research was carried out in 1998, during the course of which approximately 30,000 patients received treatment in the ED studied.

The study was part of a larger research project concerned with the way ED staff manage socially-disadvantaged patients (Fassin 1999). Fieldwork was carried out over a period of four months. It involved semi-structured interviews and field observations, which were conducted after negotiations with both the Hospital General Manager and the consultant in charge of the ED. Most of the staff of the unit were interviewed (doctors (n = 10), nurses (n = 11), auxiliaries (n = 7) and ward clerks (n = 3)). Interviews lasted between 45 minutes and one hour and a half. They were not tape-recorded. As far as was possible, hand notes were made contemporaneously in full, as is usually done in organisational ethnographies. Additionally, many spontaneous extended interview-conversations were completed. Data were also generated through the analysis of organisational documents. Observations centred on the reception function and were recorded in the form of field notes. The processing of patients was observed at various times of day and night. My research role was one of a non-participant observer. The resultant corpus of data was analysed, using an inductive approach of the kind employed in many field studies. The researcher gradually comes to discover significant classes of persons and events, their properties and their linkages, until all his/her presumed classes are displaced by those based upon observations and interviews (Schatzman and Strauss 1973).

'Re-directing' patients and rationing care

In the hospital under review ED staff refused to treat many would-be patients at the reception stage. In the language of the setting, this is usually presented as 're-directing' patients to other care settings. At interview staff argued that this did not constitute denial of care because they sent the patient to another care setting. Indeed when the patient is directed to a specialised unit in another hospital (e.g. dental ED) it is difficult to argue that staff are rationing care, because they do not have the competence to provide it. Rather, rationing takes place when the staff refuse to provide a service which they could competently provide, and when the re-directed person does not obtain the equivalent service elsewhere. The latter situation, however, may arise when the re-directed patient does not follow instructions to go to another care setting, when the care offered in that setting is not equivalent (for instance it is more expensive), or when the request for care is also refused there. When the re-direction is to the independent GPs, the risk of denial of care is high, as many patients are deterred by the cost of the consultation and as some GPs will not accept payment with vouchers for free care. In France patients can visit any doctor they choose to see, either in a hospital outpatient clinic or in a 'liberal' practice. 'Liberal' doctors are independent practitioners, be they GPs or specialists. Initially the patient pays the bill in full[1]. A percentage of the bill is then reimbursed by the state social insurance scheme, which covers almost all the population. The balance can be reimbursed by a private insurance scheme if the patient has coverage.

The control of appropriate service utilisation implies rationing of care in this ED. Building on Parker (1975 quoted by Klein *et al.* 1996), ED staff often engage in rationing by deflection; they protect their own resources by dumping the problem in the lap of other carers. The aim of this chapter is to identify the actors who make decisions at the reception stage, and to analyse the judgmental categories used to determine patient eligibility for care. These categories have four dimensions: clinical, organisational, moral, and social.

Use of clinical criteria to categorise patients

At the reception station, ED staff make a first clinical judgment about patients in interpreting signs such as the location of pain, duration and intensity of pain, and its possible origin. Using these criteria, staff distinguish between 'real emergencies' and 'non-urgent cases', which are often described in pejorative terms such as 'outpatients' and 'people who have a pain' ('personnes qui ont des bobos').

Reception clerks

The first person that most patients meet in the ED is the reception clerk. After having answered a few questions, patients are invited to give their

name and address, to present their social insurance card and to wait in a
waiting room near the reception station. The clerk registers this information
in a computer and prints it on a sheet of paper. This information will be
used by the hospital Finance Department to bill patients many months later.
The sheets are also used by the nurses, who routinely read them as they
come through from the treatment areas to collect patients to see the doctor.

In order to typify the case, reception clerks tend to ask a set of routine
questions. What is the patient's problem? Does the problem result from a
shock? (if the answer is yes, the problem is considered as a surgical case and
the person is referred to the ED surgeons). Does the person have a referral
letter from his GP? (if the answer is yes, he is immediately registered). How
long has the problem been present? According to the answers given, the
clerk may register the attending person or advise him/her to go to another
specialised ED (paediatrics ED, dental ED in another hospital etc), or to a
hospital outpatient clinic to be examined by a specialist doctor (usually an
ophthalmologist or an ENT specialist). When the clerk thinks the problem is
neither a matter for the ED, nor for the outpatient clinics, she asks a nurse
or a sister, who sometimes calls a doctor for advice.

The reception clerks, who have low social and professional status[2], complained about the difficulties of their work. There are no written guidelines,
no formalised rules. They have no clinical training and must learn the job
through their contact with other more experienced reception clerks or
nurses. At the same time they must acquire the clinical knowledge needed to
determine patients' eligibility for care, their order of precedence and their
pathways through the unit:

> At the beginning, it was not easy, I could hardly cope. It was explained to
> me: 'If it is a back pain, if the person comes on his own, he is for us (the
> medical sector of the ED). If the person has fallen, he is for surgery'. I told
> them: 'I can't ask all these questions to people, I am no doctor'. They told
> me: 'Of course, you can! You must dare to do it!' (clerk – interview).

Sometimes clerks make mistakes in the categorisation process: they confuse
what is a matter for surgery with a matter for medicine, or they fail to
recognise the clinical seriousness of a case and its urgency. According to a
general rule, patients must be processed in the order in which they arrive.
But where a patient's condition seems serious, nurses demand that the
reception clerk put their sheet on top of the pile, or at least mention the case
to them. They also want clerks to guide the most urgent cases straight
through into the unit. If reception clerks fail to do this, they are repri-
manded by nurses and doctors, something they feel is particularly unfair.
For instance, the reception clerk had given no special priority to a man who
said that he suffered tummy ache. Doctors discovered later that he had an
epigastric pain and that he was having an infarction. Conversely, the clerk
may be criticised for giving high priority to a trivial case.

The clerk's responsibilities vis-à-vis patients and the rest of the department are considerable. This confirms findings from classic studies in organisational sociology which demonstrate the crucial role played by subordinates in bureaucratic settings (Crozier 1963, Mechanic 1962), or by 'lay persons' in medical care units (Strauss *et al.* 1963). As Hughes (1989) has put it, the casualty reception clerk uses clinical categories to typify 'would-be patients'. She has no clinical expertise but she is strongly influenced by the professional culture of doctors and nurses, who delegate to her the gatekeeper role and the responsibility for prioritising patients. But many differences distinguish the British ED studied by Hughes (1989) from the French one. In the latter the clerks feel that they are not supported enough by the rest of the staff and many quit this job as soon as possible. The lack of experienced reception clerks and the greater concern to deny care to ineligible patients in this department, in comparison with the British one, mean that other staff members become more involved in the process of categorising patients at the reception station.

Nurses

In the present study, the consultant who heads the Department acknowledged the importance of the reception clerk role, although he remained unaware that informal patient categorisation sometimes implied the denial of care. He has introduced a policy that nurses should assist at the reception station, but has not introduced any formal training scheme. In practice, because of limited staff numbers, there are long periods where no nurse is present behind the desk. Moreover, nurses dislike undertaking this task, which they find unrewarding. Like the clerks, they have received no specific training, and the job is not clearly defined. Typically, the clerk calls a nurse when she believes one is needed. Nurses acknowledge that they work 'each one in her own way': the only informal rule is to call the doctor when in doubt or when the patient refuses to be 're-directed' elsewhere. Some doctors question nurses' abilities to screen attenders, and take the view that only they should make decisions to re-direct patients. But other clinicians recognise that nurses must be involved in patient categorisation, delegate this role to them and intervene only if the would-be patient insists on seeing a doctor.

It is not for the nurse to make the decision whether the patient should be admitted here or not. Doing a diagnosis with only a few elements is difficult. It is even more difficult for a nurse. (...) When the nurse is embarrassed, she goes looking for a doctor (doctor A – interview).

It is the reception nurse who usually tells them (the attending persons) that their problem is not so serious. The guy says: 'Yeah, I want to see the doctor!' The doctor comes and says the same thing. Nurses sometimes make a boob, but it's rare (doctor B – interview).

In categorising patients, the nurse starts with much the same questions as the reception clerk. What is the problem you came for? For how long has it lasted? How did it happen? But she then asks more precise clinical questions to get additional information about the symptoms and the possible origins of the problem. Depending on the information received, the nurse has a number of options. She may authorise the clerk to register the attending person, she may advise that person to consult a doctor in another hospital setting (specialised ED, outpatients clinics with an immediate or postponed appointment), or she may call a doctor to get him/her to persuade the person to consult an outside doctor (GP, psychological care centre, people's dispensary, etc.).

One of the main criteria used by nurses to determine patients' eligibility for care was the duration of the problem. Most staff operate on the basis that if the problem has lasted for more than a few days, they consider that it is not a emergency condition. For instance, a reception nurse tried to convince a man in his 50s, talking with a Hispanic accent, to go to consult a GP. This man said he had back pain from a work accident which happened one month previously. He argued that he did not want to see a GP because this doctor would send him to the pharmacist and to the (independent) radiologist. It would take him time and money. The nurse called a doctor who denied him care and advised him to see a GP.

Doctors
Several ED doctors, including the senior consultant and his deputy, considered that only 15 to 20 per cent of attenders are 'real emergencies' or 'really urgent cases'. Whatever their professional status and length of service[3], all ED doctors agreed that cases like this, which involved a risk to life, had a legitimate claim to treatment. They quoted serious asthma, cardiac infarction, acute lung oedema and multiple-injuries as examples. They also emphasised the need to examine patients who presented unclear symptoms where diagnosis was uncertain but potentially grave, for example: headache, thoracic pain and abdominal pain. At interview they all eventually discussed 'outpatients', namely patients presenting with minor health problems, which are not appropriate for the ED. However, they differed in their opinions about whether all cases of this kind warranted clinical examination.

The senior consultant and his deputy both maintained that every person attending the department was examined by a doctor. They explained that it was impossible to know if the patient had a serious condition without examining him as part of a detailed consultation, and underlined their medical and legal accountability. The other practitioners could be divided into two groups. In the language of the setting, the 'broad ones' examine every attending person, or most of them. In their opinion, the public hospital as an institution has a responsibility to provide care to all those who need it. They also underlined the risk of medical mistakes if the provisional diagnosis made at the reception station was wrong. They gave numerous instances of the difficulties in using these clinical criteria, at first glance, without examining the patient.

Conversely the 'firm ones' re-direct most attenders whose cases seem to be trivial. They felt that, if the health problem was minor or had lasted for a few days, the attender could wait a few hours more to access the health care system via a different route. A 'firm' doctor had denied care to a man in his 30s, who suffered insomnia. This attender explained that he had not slept well for three months, mentioning his work on the nightshift and some family problems. He also mentioned that he had been helped out a few times in this ED and that he would like to have tranquillisers. The doctor told him to go and see a GP in his local area who would refer him, if necessary, to a Psychological Care Centre.

The 'firm' doctors asserted that if staff treat attenders with minor conditions, they risk not having enough time and human resources to diagnose and treat patients with serious health problems. Other complex arguments were presented. The main argument relates to what is best for the patients in the long run: to get disadvantaged patients into the habit of coming to the ED is not good for them; they would be better off looking for a doctor in a health care setting who can provide both initial treatment and continuing care. What is at stake is to educate the patients as to how they should use the health system. Other arguments are related to the division of labour in the health care system: free care in ED amounts to unfair competition with independent GPs located in the same area. Moreover, the real cost to the social insurance scheme of hospital care for a benign pathology is higher than the cost in most community-based health care settings.

Doctors acknowledged that their practices differed and that there was little prospect of change for the moment:

Some doctors think that they can educate the clientele: 'This is an outpatient case' and they turn it away to the GP. I myself am much less firm. Behaviours are not consistent. (. . .) The doctor's personality plays a big role. Some of them open the umbrella, as we say in our jargon, and some of them say: 'This is an outpatient case, and the Outpatients Clinic will send him back to us if this is grave' (doctor A – interview).

These disagreements within the medical team were well known to other staff, from the reception clerks and auxiliaries to the nursing sister. Staff explained that 'you have to adapt yourself to the psychology of each doctor'. When the doctor in charge is a 'broad' one, receptionists and nurses register all attending persons. When he is a 'firm' doctor, staff generally call him to see the most contentious cases, but also appear to exercise more discretion in re-directing minor cases to other agencies or independent GPs. Different doctors fall along a continuum from the 'broadest' to the 'firmest'.

But even 'broad doctors' may exceptionally be firm with an attender and vice versa. Doctors distinguished between legitimate and illegitimate attenders, using criteria that were not exclusively clinical.

Use of organisational criteria to categorise patients

These criteria are not related to the attributes of the presenting patient, but to the characteristics of the unit at the time of attendance. Depending on the number of patients present in the waiting room, the reception clerk may re-direct more or fewer attenders to other care settings:

> We decide whether to register her or him (an attender presenting with a minor health problem), depending on the physical state of the patient, depending on the staff workload or on the length of the queue (sister – interview).

Other factors specific to the organisation of this hospital play a role in the registration decision. For example, because the on-call psychiatrist arrives only in the evening and is not available during the day, patients with suspected psychiatric disorders (such as the one mentioned above) are often redirected elsewhere. Similarly, the extent of co-operation between the ED and different hospital outpatient clinics is an important consideration. Outpatient clinic staff will say over the telephone whether appointment slots are available for patients who could be re-directed to them. If no appointments are available the case is likely to be processed in the ED. In certain clinics, like ENT, staff rarely offer appointments. As a consequence, the reception clerks register more patients with the type of pathology referred to such clinics compared with conditions treatable in clinics where appointments are available.

Additionally, as Roth (1972) and Roth and Douglas (1983) suggest, the general organisation of the national health care system plays a role. The day and the time of patient arrival determines whether re-direction is possible or not, depending on the availability of other health professionals and facilities. For example, outpatient clinics in this hospital are open only on weekdays from 9.00 a.m. to 4.00 p.m. During the evening and at the weekend, emergency staff only rarely re-direct patients, and during the night they never do.

Use of moral criteria to categorise patients

Just as described by Roth (1972) and Roth and Douglas (1983), ED staff express moral judgements about people attending the department. In the French ED, these moral evaluations can influence the registration decision, the order of precedence amongst patients, and staff behaviour towards them. In this chapter, I have space to document only two forms of evaluation which may influence the registration decisions – concerned with staff perceptions that patients use the unit for their own 'convenience' and must respect previous instructions.

In the study hospital, when patients present with conditions that staff consider trivial, and openly state that they have come to the ED because it is more convenient than other health care settings, they are very likely to be re-directed elsewhere. ED staff were unanimous in rejecting the idea that the hospital was merely the provider of a technical service, offering quicker treatments and more convenient opening hours than other health care settings. The case of a patient with the 'industrial injury' mentioned above illustrates the negative reaction incurred by patients who are perceived to be making demands on the service for their own convenience. A further example is that reception clerks have been instructed to re-direct persons who come to the ED to get a second medical opinion, after having consulted another doctor for the same condition.

Staff also expressed disapproval of patients who fail to follow instructions about return visits to the hospital. Patients who return frequently to the ED seeking treatment for minor conditions break an unwritten rule about the proper demands they can make. In the example of the attender with insomnia, the doctor on duty justified his decision to deny care by underlining the fact that the patient had mentioned several previous visits to the department. This argument worked against him. The doctor considered that he had to redirect the patient for his own good. Another rule, which is explicit, forbids patients to come back for a number of specific treatments, such as changing bandages, removing sutures, and checking plaster casts. ED staff re-direct persons needing these services to the outpatients clinics.

Use of social criteria to categorise patients

ED staff have constructed an informal system for rationing care for patients with minor ailments. However, they attenuate the rationing according to the attender's social situation.

Lack of knowledge of the health care system

ED staff routinely attempted to assess the extent to which individual patients were acquainted with the French care system. They wanted to know whether the attending patient possessed the cognitive, psychological and linguistic resources that would enable him/her to identify an alternative source of care and to explain his/her health problems. If staff thought that the patient was unable to do so, they were more likely to allow registration in the ED. They often assumed that foreigners had an inadequate knowledge of the system:

There are always cases where a reception nurse catches somebody who has not got proper social security. This person does not speak French well, looks completely lost and has not been in France for long. I register these people without even asking the doctor. It is our job to do this. If the doctor asks me 'why did you register this woman?' I reply: 'because this is our job!' (nurse – interview).

A reception clerk or nurse noticing a patient's lack of familiarity with the health care system might be influenced in favour of registration. However, this would not be seen as giving sufficient grounds in all cases. In cases where a patient is re-directed, the effects of denying immediate treatment can be softened. For instance, the nurse may telephone the doctor in charge of the service to which the patient has been referred to make the appointment.

Recognisable social problems

Staff often make judgements about the economic resources of patients. A presumption that the patient is poor is conducive to registration. Members of staff recognise that those experiencing social problems probably lack the resources to pay an independent GP:

We try to convince attending persons suffering minor ailments to go and see a GP, except in some cases where we have to see them against our will. This happens during weekends and with people suffering from deprivation. They tell us 'Yes, you are right, but I do not have enough to pay' (doctor C – interview).

The most extreme case is that of homeless people. This is the type of case that staff immediately mention when asked about people so disadvantaged that they may have no other access to medical care. Staff assert that a number of homeless people attend the emergency service on a regular basis, if only to have an opportunity to eat and sleep. The homeless people who attend the service are not re-directed.

ED staff assess presenting patients on multiple dimensions, which often point in the same direction. Thus, a patient who has little familiarity with the health care system, who is seen to be poor and has social problems (such as isolation or family difficulties) is more likely to be registered. A 'broad' doctor had agreed to see a 30-year-old who had 'flu', on the basis that he was living on his own, worked as a cleaner, did not speak French fluently and had missed his appointment at the social dispensary. Similarly, a nurse registered a woman who said she had been coughing for two weeks and then mentioned domestic violence problems.

Members of staff did sometimes re-direct individuals seen to have social problems. They usually, however, took this factor into account when choosing the health services to which these individuals were re-directed, mostly social dispensaries. The nurses also smooth the way for the patient by making a call to arrange the appointment with a dispensary or a GP.

Having no family doctor
ED staff considered whether the would-be patient has a family doctor or not. They assumed that it was relatively easy for patients with a GP to gain access to an alternative source of care and were likely to steer them in that direction. Those who had no GP might get a more sympathetic reception. The 'firmer' doctors, however, refused to consider this issue. As shown in the example of the patient requesting tranquillisers, they sought to discourage patients from acquiring the 'habit' of attending emergency services for minor health problems. In many such cases, re-directing the patient meant advising him/her to look for a GP in his/her area, who would become his/her family doctor.

> People are re-directed toward a GP only when we are confident that they can afford to go there. They tell us they 'don't know anybody'. We tell them that this is precisely the time when they should attempt to get to know somebody. This is not denying care, it is rather educating the patient (doctor B – interview).

The lack of social security entitlements
The hospital Finance Director had instructed administrative and health care staff to ask patients to present a social security card as soon as they arrived in the ED. If they did not have one, they were to present an identity card. As confirmed by my observations, however, the consensus among the staff was that the absence of social security entitlements, or documents entitling the individual to stay in France, should not preclude the registration of patients. It is a fact that the clerks ask for a social security card or, if the patient does not have one, an identity card. They nevertheless register the patient even if he/she cannot produce these documents. In such cases the registration details are based on the information given orally by the patient.

Many staff saw this as a positive reflection of their social obligations. They strenuously denounced other hospitals and clinics in the area, which denied access to care on the basis of such criteria. They suggested that lack of social security entitlements in this ED might help justify registration, even when the condition was relatively trivial. This contrasts with the attitude taken towards patients who have the correct social security documents, and who could go elsewhere.

Discussion and conclusion

In this ED some staff perceived the rationing of care as a strategy for coping with growing demand in the context of limited human resources. As they interact together they elaborate informal rules concerning the eligibility and priority of patients for treatment in the ED. Their decision making cannot be analysed as a purely bureaucratic process, based on the application of procedural rules. Neither can it be analysed as a typical street-level bureaucracy in which staff interpret the existing protocols, since no written procedures exist in this ED. The law states that all attenders must be seen, but it does not specify the nature of the clinical assessment[4].

In this chapter I have described the various criteria used by ED staff to categorise patients, and the way they combined these criteria, using the approach developed by Elster and Herpin (Elster 1992, Elster and Herpin 1992). The clinical criterion was always given priority in deciding whether or not to register a patient. Attenders with minor health problems were likely to be re-directed at the reception station. But other criteria might also come into play.

As found in earlier ED studies, organisational and moral criteria were also taken into account in the decisions concerning the registration of patients. Staff re-directed patients to other health care settings only during normal opening hours (not in the evening, at night or during the weekend) and only when there was a queue in the ward. Often they arrived at a negative moral judgement on the attenders openly stating that they had come to the ED because it was more convenient for them, or saying that they wanted a second medical opinion. If, in addition, the patient had a minor condition, he or she was likely to be turned away.

Finally, judgements about patients' eligibility were influenced by assessments of their social situation. Staff tended to follow an informal rule according to which they accepted persons with social problems or lack of knowledge of the health system, whatever the clinical seriousness of their condition. In effect, they had set up an informal system of positive discrimination[5]. By doing so, they construct a noble image of themselves as caring public servants. These data are at odds with Roth's and Jeffery's findings, which indicate that staff favoured patients seen as having high social value. There are several possible explanations for these different findings. First, they may be related to differences in the socio-economic background of the countries and periods studied (Dodier and Camus 1998). In the French ED, staff members tried to construct the meaning of their work as a response to the consequences of the perceived economic and social crisis of the late 1990s. Second, this general hospital is located in a deprived Parisian suburb and lacks the prestige of teaching hospitals. Some doctors who worked in this ED originate from deprived immigrant backgrounds. They might feel closer to disadvantaged patients than to those from middle class backgrounds. Finally the different results may relate in part to the different research methods used. This research relied as much on interviews as on observational data. Interviews provide a way of accessing the criteria used by the staff when they make decisions related to patients' eligibility for care, and in so doing, they illuminate the factors that influence admission to the ED.

The present study suggests some new insights into the nature of categorisation. ED staff categorised patients and consequently accepted, refused or speeded up the processing of presenting cases. Yet, in comparison with previous ED studies, the analysis of the rules used by the staff to build these categories shows that their behaviour cannot be interpreted only as deriving from the drive to 'professionalize' their occupation. Building on Elster (1992), I consider that staff created two 'local theories of justice' to allocate limited human resources in a way they perceived to be equitable. One is based on an egalitarian ideal (to give each patient the same service). Thus 'broad' doctors tend to admit all attenders. The second theory of justice is based on an ideal of equity (to give each patient the services s/he needs). Thus 'firm' doctors deny registration to individuals with benign problems. But people considered to be poor are less likely to be turned away. Taking into account the fact that this ED accepts a larger proportion of disadvantaged patients than most other public or private hospitals, these doctors formulate a new version of the public service ethos. The hospital's mission is not to welcome everybody and as a consequence to provide 'comfort medicine' to middle class patients; rather, it is to treat deprived patients who do not have access to care elsewhere.

Many ED doctors considered that this positive discrimination in favour of the socially disadvantaged, exempted them from criticism. They thought that they had the right and the competence to judge patients' needs. This categorisation of patients, however, leads to the micro-rationing of care because it is likely that some patients who have been re-directed will not obtain the equivalent service in another health care facility. Some of them may even not see any doctor at all. Moreover, in searching for equity, doctors sacrifice the ideal of impartiality, according to which different people receive equal treatment according to need. Many ethicists argue that where differing treatments are provided for different groups, this should be based on principles which are applied consistently to everybody (Elster 1992). But in this ED, a person with a given non-urgent condition who is registered one day could be refused the day after, according to such factors as the doctor in charge, the number queuing in the waiting room, and the interpretation made of his or her social situation.

The underlying conception of distributive justice recognised in this setting is negotiated between various actors, who have more or less legitimate authority to fix the rules. The reception clerk is not authorised to determine patients' eligibility. When she detects certain characteristics in the case of the presenting person, she has to call for a nurse or a doctor, who will decide whether to accept the attender or not. She has more room for manoeuvre in determining patients' order of precedence. Some nurses take responsibility for making decisions to accept patients, but most ask the doctor to make the decision. Where nurses take on this role, it is often because they are working with doctors who have indicated their willingness to delegate this task to the individual involved. Only doctors can decide which models of local justice will be taken into account. Two distinct models can be distinguished in this ED because two groups of doctors with the same hierarchical status disagree on what to do, and a senior consultant (who is distanced from the daily life of the ED) allows them to determine policy on a case-by-case basis. This research shows that our understanding of the patient categorisation process must not be limited to the study of the interactions between would-be patients and the reception staff. It must be backed up with the analysis of power relations between staff members, who elaborate, fix and change the local informal rules in a dynamic process.

Acknowledgments

I am grateful to Davina Allen, Hervé Hudebine, David Hughes, Marc Robert and one anonymous reviewer for their helpful comments on earlier drafts of this chapter.

Notes

1 The exception may be patients who have vouchers for free care. Local Authorities distribute these vouchers to low-income residents deemed eligible, but some independent practitioners do not accept payment with vouchers.

2 The reception clerks are employees of the Admissions Department, which administers the recovery of patient invoice charges. Four members of staff share this job every day from 07.00 to 23.00 hrs. They are all young and have a limited education. Their professional status is lower than that of other hospital civil servants, they are on fixed-term contracts, in some cases part-time, and their wages are low. Three of them are women. Two of them live in the social housing blocks surrounding the hospital. 18 months into the study, two of the four had moved to other clerical posts in the hospital.

3 The medical team includes a consultant in charge of the Department, three other senior doctors ('praticiens hospitaliers'), four doctors equivalent to Senior Registrar ('médecins assistants'), four general practitioners who work part time in the Emergency Department and three Health Officers. The turn-over is high (of 12 doctors working in this unit in 1997, only five still worked here one year after).

4 This is from 'loi du 31 juillet 1991 portant réforme hospitalière'. See also the 'Circulaire du 21 mars 1995 relative à l'accès aux soins des personnes les plus démunies' du Ministère des Affaires Sociales. See also the 'Code de la Santé Publique' (article L711-4) which mentions that 'hospitals are open to every individual whose condition requires their service. They must be able to welcome them night and day, if necessary urgently'.

5 These data are supported by the findings of social scientists studying other French street-level bureaucracies, such as Family Allowance Departments (Dubois 1999) or Social Housing Offices (Weller 1998a), which show that, against the background of the economic crisis of the 1990s, civil servants often exercised discretion to favour deprived people. These sociological studies also underline the fact that the analysis of public sector work and the public service ethos needs to be placed in a wider social and political context (Weller 1998b).

References

Crozier, M. (1963) *Le phénomène bureaucratique*. Paris: Seuil.

Crozier, M. and Friedberg, E. (1977) *L'acteur et le système*. Paris: Seuil.

Dodier, N. and Camus, A. (1998) Openness and specialisation: dealing with patients in a hospital emergency service, *Sociology of Health and Illness*, 20, 413–44.

Dubois, V. (1999) *La vie au guichet*. Paris, Economica.

Elster, J. (1992) *Local Justice*. Cambridge: Cambridge University Press.

Elster, J. and Herpin, N. (1992) *Ethique des choix médicaux*. Arles: Actes Sud.

Fassin, D. (1999) *Les Urgences et la précarité*. Université Paris XIII-Bobigny: Rapport du Centre de Recherche sur les Enjeux de Santé Publique.

Glaser, B. and Strauss, A. (1965) *Awareness of Dying*. Chicago: Aldine.

Griffiths, L. and Hughes, D. (1994) 'Innocent parties' and 'disheartening' experiences: natural rhetorics in neuro-rehabilitation admissions conferences, *Qualitative Health Research*, 4, 385–410.

Hoffman, J.E. (1974) 'Nothing can be done': Social dimensions of the treatment of stroke patients in a general hospital, *Urban Life and Culture*, 3, 50–70.

Hughes, D. (1989) Paper and people: the work of the casualty reception clerk, *Sociology of Health and Illness*, 11, 382–408.

Hughes, E.C. (1971) *The Sociological Eye*. Chicago: Aldine-Atherton.

Jeffery, R. (1979) Normal rubbish: deviant patients in casualty departments. *Sociology of Health and Illness*, 1, 90–107.

Kelly, M.P. and May, D. (1982) Good and bad patients: a review of the literature and a theoretical critique, *Journal of Advanced Nursing*, 7, 147–56.

Klein, R., Day, P. and Redmayne, S. (1996) *Managing Scarcity: Priority Setting and Rationing in the National Health Service*. Buckingham: Open University Press.

Lorber, J. (1975) Good patients and problem patients: conformity and deviance in a general hospital, *Journal of Health and Social Behaviour*, 16, 213–25.

Mannon, J.M. (1976) Defining and treating 'problem' patients in a hospital emergency setting, *Medical Care*, 14, 1004–13.

May, D. and Kelly, M.P. (1982) 'Chancers, pests and poor wee souls': problems of legitimation in psychiatric nursing, *Sociology of Health and Illness*, 4, 279–97.

Mechanic, D. (1962) Sources of power of lower participants in complex organizations, *Administrative Science Quarterly*, 7, 349–64.

Roth, J.A. (1972) Some contingencies of the moral evaluation and control of clientele: the case of the hospital emergency service, *American Journal of Sociology*, 77, 839–57.

Roth, J.A. and Douglas, D. (1983) *No Appointment Necessary*. New York: Irvington.

Schatzman, L. and Strauss, A.L. (1973) *Field Research. Strategies for a Natural Sociology*. Englewood Cliffs: Prentice Hall.

Strauss, A.L., Schatzman, L., Ehrlich, D., Bucher, R. and Sabshin, M. (1963) The hospital and its negotiated order. In Freidson, E. (ed) *The Hospital in Modern Society*. New York: The Free Press.

Sudnow, D. (1967) *Passing On*. Englewood Cliffs, New Jersey: Prentice Hall Inc.

Sudnow, D. (1973) Dead on arrival. In Strauss, A. (ed) *When Medicine Fails*. New Brunswick: Transaction Books.

Timmermans, S. (1999) *Sudden Death and the Myth of CPR*. Philadelphia: Temple University Press.

Vassy, C. (1999) Travailler à l'hôpital en Europe. *Revue Française de Sociologie*, 40, 325–56.

Weller, J.M. (1998a) *Le bureaucrate et l'usager*. Paris: Desclée de Brouwer.

Weller, J.M. (1998b) La modernisation des services publics par l'usager, *Sociologie du Travail*, 3, 365–92.

Wolcott, B.W. (1979) What is an emergency? Depends on whom you ask, *Journal of American College of Emergency Physicians*, 8, 241–3.

5

Everyday experiences of implicit rationing: comparing the voices of nurses in California and British Columbia

Ivy Lynn Bourgeault, Pat Armstrong, Hugh Armstrong, Jacqueline Choiniere, Joel Lexchin, Eric Mykhalovskiy, Suzanne Peters and Jerry White

Introduction

Rationing health care to curb rising costs is a complex, politically charged issue. This is no less true for the country with the highest percentage of health care spending measured as a percentage of Gross Domestic Product (GDP), the U.S. at 14.4 per cent, or Canada that spends 10.1 per cent of GDP (Armstrong and Armstrong 1996: 165). Indeed, analysts in the U.S. argue that rationing is the pre-eminent health policy issue of the 1990s (Conrad and Brown 1993). In Canada, although the debate over health care reform has not focused explicitly on rationing per se, poll after poll has shown that overall cutbacks to health care, which implicitly involves rationing, is the primary concern citizens.

Rationing of care comes in a variety of forms. Mariner (1995) describes the traditional distinction between the more implicit, upstream forms of rationing, or *macro*allocation, that include government policy, funding decisions, and distribution of services; and the more explicit, downstream rationing, or *micro*allocation, that occurs at patients' bedside. Much of the debate around rationing of care is centred on macroallocation policies and is often discussed in terms of principles of social justice, moral rights and societal responsibilities (*c.f.* Blake 1994, Daniels 1985, Daniels *et al.* 1996, Goold 1996, Light 1999). More recently, however, research has increasingly focused on the methods by which physicians allocate at the bedside (Ubel and Goold 1997, Bloomfield 1991). Daniels (1986), for example, reports that physicians in the U.S. find rationing decisions difficult and unfair because they cannot point to a just macroallocation scheme that justifies denying care to patients. Studies in the U.K., by contrast, have found that simple notions of cost-effectiveness in clinical decision making are accepted by most GPs. They do, however, report increasing pressure from patient demand, rising stress and declining morale (Baines *et al.* 1998).

Physicians and other health care providers are not, however, simply the passive agents of rationing policies. Hughes and Griffiths (1996, 1997), for example, highlight the agency of physicians in the U.K. in micro resource allocations decisions. Such decisions often rest on social or moral judgements about patients' characteristics. Timmermans' (1999) investigation of resuscitative efforts also reveals how the presumed social worth of the patients plays an important role in the implicit rationing of lifesaving endeavours by emergency department staff. Light (1999) argues similarly that physicians in Canada exercise a great deal of relatively unaccountable discretion in the practice of rationing through waiting lists.

Between macro and microallocation decisions lie institutional and organisational decisions – which could be referred to as *meso*allocation – that equally affect access to care by individual patients (Mariner 1995). Here one could include the increasing usage of clinical guidelines or evidence-based practice (EBP) which some have argued can help minimise bedside rationing (Grimshaw and Hutchinson 1995, Klein *et al.* 1996). EBP could also, however, be viewed as a form of rationing in and of itself. Indeed, according to Orentlicher (1998), one of the myths associated with practice guidelines is that they can avert the need for physicians to make coverage decisions at the bedside.

One of the most recent methods of rationing health care that could be situated at the *meso* level and that involves tacit rationing, is the application of what are promoted as new managerial strategies for health care, borrowed in large part from the private sector. Specifically called *Managed Care*[1] in the U.S., these methods have been creeping into other countries, including Canada, where certain kinds of care are similarly being 'managed', albeit in a different socio-political context. The overall goal of these implicit rationing strategies is to do more with less; the promise is better health care at a cheaper cost. In the U.S., rationing decisions are made primarily in the private sector[2] with each organisation freely applying its own criteria to ration health care resulting in a multitude of coverage plans (Mariner 1995, McMillan 1993). Because of its location in the private sector little is known about how these decisions are made. The result has been an exacerbation of the longstanding issue of lack of accessibility – or the problem of the *uninsured* – and the growing problem of the *underinsured* (Carrasquillo *et al.* 1999)[3].

In Canada, where, as in the U.K., universality and accessibility are key principles built into the organisation of government-funded health care, rationing affects not so much access to care as timing (*i.e.* how long one has to wait to get care), and the amount of care. Generally speaking, access is guaranteed within a certain period of time; however, the length of this waiting period still varies widely by geography and other social demographic variables, even if somewhat less so than in the U.S. (Armstrong and Armstrong 1998a).

Guaranteed access is not the only issue that differentiates the U.S. and Canadian health care systems. Analysts argue that they are fundamentally different systems built on a different set of principles and logic. Tuohy (1999), for example, highlights the fact that in Canada, coverage is of *services*, whereas in the U.S. coverage is of *individuals*. In Canada there is universal access to funded services, whereas in the U.S. there is restricted access for funded individuals. In turn, the focus of rationing in the U.S. is on the insured person, whereas in Canada rationing initiatives focus on insured services.

In this chapter, we examine from a comparative perspective the rationing of health care in the U.S. and Canada drawing on the experiences of nurses in California and British Columbia (B.C.). We focus on nurses primarily because it is they who have regular and prolonged contact with patients and provide the bulk of health care within this 'managed' system. They, therefore, are in an excellent position to describe the practices of rationing and their impact on both patients and providers. Despite the important perspective nurses have of the practice of rationing, there has been little empirical research published, particularly from a comparative perspective. Most of the empirical literature examines physicians' views and experiences. Where the nursing perspective is considered, it usually entails an editorial rather than an empirical analysis of the need for rationing (Davis 1991, Huey 1990, Mittelstadt 1985, Reigle 1990, Stevens 1992), its inevitability (Andrews 1993, Hancock 1993, Perrin 1989, Wells 1995), and the ethical dilemmas it presents nurses (Coombs 1990).

The research we present here could initially be considered to be a micro level of analysis. We argue, however, as we have in our previous work as a group, that the micro experiences of health care providers cannot be divorced from the meso context of managerial strategies – in this case aimed at rationing care (Armstrong and Armstrong 1996). What we find in this research is that the price to be paid for the promise of better, cheaper health care is conspicuous in the voices of nurses working on both sides of the border. Rationing of care under Managed Care in the U.S. and similar methods of 'managing' care in Canada, as filtered through the interpretive lens of nurses, does not deliver on its claims of more appropriate or more affordable health care. Indeed, nurses argue that they and other health care providers bear the brunt of any cost savings associated with the increased management of care. What also becomes apparent from our comparative analysis is that although nurses in B.C. and California share similar experiences and complaints with the application of managerial strategies to health care, their experiences are shaped by the different socio-political contexts of the health care system within which they work.

Methods

Nine mixed group interviews were conducted in California in September 1997 with 35 Registered Nurses employed in a variety of Managed Care settings. Purposive sampling was employed to ensure a range of nursing experiences with Managed Care. Nurse participants worked in intensive care units in hospitals and public health units in communities, general medical/surgical wards and advice nursing, home health and emergency rooms, outpatient surgery and as nurse practitioners in Health Maintenance Organisations (HMOs). To contrast the data on nurses' Managed Care experience in California, 10 mixed group interviews were conducted one month later in B.C., Canada with 39 Registered Nurses employed in a similar range of settings to those noted for the California nurses.

Participation in both sets of interviews was fully consensual. In a typical case, three to five nurses would spend two or more hours in a neutral location separate from their places of work discussing with two of the authors how health care was being managed. Interviews were largely conversational with questioning loosely following the main claims of Managed Care we set out to address: namely, integration and continuity; accountability for appropriate care; and health promotion and disease prevention. All interviews were tape-recorded, transcribed verbatim and thematically coded for analysis along these claims. Rationing of care emerged as a critical theme from the accounts of nurses in both settings. That is, our focus here on the issue of rationing forms a sort of secondary data analysis; we did not directly ask nurses about their views on rationing per se but in their responses to the issue of the management of care they spoke volumes of the implicit rationing of both the *access* to various forms of care and of the *amount* of care patients received once they had gained access to the system.

Rationing access to care: *denying and delaying*

Do anything you can to prevent them from coming in (CA Grp 5).

An implicit form of rationing care involves limiting access to various forms of care. Based on our interviews with nurses, we found this to be accomplished primarily by *denying* access in the California case and *delaying* access in the B.C. case.

Accessing acute care
All the ways in which citizens access acute health care in California – insurers, public clinics and hospital Emergency Rooms (ERs) – have increasingly experienced rationing, and the consequences of this become quite

clear in the California nurses' interviews. For example, under Managed Care, there is increasing pressure on patients and physicians in Health Maintenance Organisations (HMOs) to reduce expenditures, and cost reduction begins in the doctor's office. This means 'people don't go see the doctors as frequently as they used to because ... insurance won't pay' (CA Grp 4). Physicians, operating under strict rules, also deny care, as one nurse said:

> I'm seeing physicians under capitation who will not send patients to the
> hospital in times where they used to ... because the physicians' ...
> contracts or whatever with the HMOs or Managed Care organisations,
> are saying, 'Well, you can't go over a certain amount of money' (CA Grp 4).

Nurses in California also told stories about denial of care by insurance companies:

> They go to the doctor and the doctor makes a referral to the insurance
> company. ... And then you fight with this high school person on a
> computer [at the insurance company] that says this person with that
> diagnosis doesn't need this [care] (CA Grp 7).

Care is not only rationed once the physician is seen, in many cases access is limited through various barriers set up before patients can see a physician. One example of this is the increasing use of nurse-staffed Call Centres that patients must call before they can get to see a physician. Their main purpose, according to these nurses, is to prevent people from coming in.

Access to care is also limited at public clinics because there are so few of them and, where they do exist, there are extensive waiting times. Patients who finally gain access care at these clinics may have to see whatever physician is available; and the physician they do get acts as a 'gatekeeper', limiting or denying care similar to physicians in HMOs.

Another point of access, and often the only point for many California citizens, are ERs. According to nurses here, patients often come to the ER either because they do not have a primary care doctor, or because they cannot get care in any other way, even from their own primary care physician:

> If they call on the phone, they might wait an hour or a half hour before
> somebody talks to them on the phone ... They think if they come to the
> emergency room it'll be faster (CA Grp 3).

Indeed, newly-passed government legislation requires that everyone who comes to the ER must be assessed; thus, emergency care cannot be rationed by exclusions based on finances or coverage. In some cases nurses tell of how they circumvent the denial of care in hospital by whispering to patients to check themselves in through the ER:

[You say] 'Yes, your procedure has been denied and I know you're in absolute agony now. But you could always leave the hospital and go to the emergency room'. Or if you need to be seen 'I know you are hurting in your stomach but say you have chest pains and you'll get seen rapidly' (CA Grp 9).

But even in the ER, patients are denied care:

Frequently I'm hearing stories from people who it takes three or four visits to the emergency room before they get admitted to the hospital.... They're coming back so much sicker ... or are going home and dying (CA Grp 4).

In the case of access to emergency care, the denial of care California nurses talk about is similar to B.C. nurses' accounts of the delaying of care. In B.C., rationing in ERs results from closures, amalgamations and the movement toward reducing duplication of services. Nurses in B.C. tell of some distressing situations that have arisen in the transition period:

They closed the neuro at [hospital A] and put it over at [hospital B] and they kept no neuro instruments at [hospital A] so an ambulance who's told ... to go to the closest hospital ... with some poor head injury ... Well we couldn't do anything ... We didn't have any neuro instruments. And they had to put her back in the ambulance and drive her all the way across town. ... She died (BC Grp 1).

Generally speaking, however, these cases of the denial of care arising from the reduction in services are rare in B.C. and nurses there did not experience the kinds of day-to-day denial of care that California nurses told about in story after story. In the case of accessing preventive care, we also found notable differences between California and B.C. nurses' experience.

Accessing preventive care
In recent years HMOs have claimed significant improvements in preventive care aimed at keeping their members healthy. Under Managed Care, however, this focus has shifted toward short-term cost containment. For example, nurses noted the demise of annual physical examinations and how one HMO ...

has a 50 year history of health prevention and ... going to a physical ... That's been cut out. ... They don't encourage it. They issued out this book instead, and ... you should have already looked in that book to see what you could have done to avoid your coming into the emergency room, the clinic, or even making that call. That's their ... idea [of prevention] (CA Grp 3).

Nurses point out how increasingly appointments are allowed only if a problem has already developed, and are so brief that it is extremely unlikely that any assessment of the whole person will be done. Perhaps more importantly for those on limited budgets, appointments now usually involve a cost, or co-payment, even when the service is covered under the Managed Care plan:

> You used to have free office results. Now you're going to have to pay a $10 co-pay. ... [and] there's more exclusions to what's covered (CA Grp 5).

As a result, people may not get care until their illness has become severe.

Like the physical, other tests designed to allow early intervention have become less frequent. Pap smears, for example, are not done 'annually anymore; every other year is good enough' (CA Grp 3). Others have moved to 'every three years' (CA Grp 4)[4]. Mammograms offer yet another example, where 'you have to wait on a waiting list to even get into the women's health department to be seen, then they tell you whether they're even going to order it or not' (CA Grp 5). There are also 'no prostate cancer blood tests' (CA Grp 4) covered by Managed Care plans. Non-medical prevention strategies are even less likely to be covered.

> [You can] get mammograms and pap smears, but well baby care – no – you pay for that out of pocket (CA Grp 4).

According to these nurses, Managed Care in California seems to be more about promoting profits and preventing health or as one nurse put it, 'Managed Care ... prevents care' (CA Grp 9). This is exacerbated by the constant mergers and amalgamations of Managed Care organisations leaving little incentive to invest in patients' health over the long term.

By way of contrast, nurses in B.C. have very little to recount about the shift in focus away from preventive health measures:

> Everybody here gets [immunisations] automatically for free and we even do hepatitis B now [for] all of the kids up to grade 12 (BC Grp 4).

Indeed, with recent health care reform initiatives, such as regionalisation, which were just beginning to be implemented at the time of the interviews, there was a hope that there would be an even greater shift in focus toward health promotion and the social determinants of health. Moreover, when nurses in California spoke of health promotion and preventive medicine, the discussion was in the very limited terms of disease screening tests and immunisations, whereas in B.C., the nurses had a much broader definition of health promotion. There are, for example, preventive health nursing offices that cover a range of problems, and gerontology, wellness, and addiction clinics that seek to address a range of public health issues. As one nurse who worked at one such clinic explained:

Most of my time is spent teaching and counselling community development and that's what I think of as health promotion (BC Grp 2).

Thus, we find here too a fundamental difference in the impact of rationing initiatives on access to care in the two settings.

Accessing chronic and palliative care
The rationing of access to care that nurses describe in California is not limited to acute and preventive care. Nurses also tell of how chronically ill and elderly patients are specific targets of rationing care schemes under Managed Care. As one nurse explained:

They're targeting certain groups, especially people that are chronically ill and they're calling those the high users. And they're identifying these people that over-utilize the system ... now they're trying to figure out ways to keep them from coming in (CA Grp 5).

One practice that this nurse describes, is to 'make them go to group classes so that you don't even get to see a physician; you don't get any individual care' (CA Grp 5). Another strategy involves arbitrarily limiting the number of home or office visits a patient can have, regardless of the complexity of his or her case:

[The organisation] said, 'let's trim all our visits down to 10. Ten is going to be the average number of visits, no matter what'. ... there are a lot of cases that are fairly simple, that can be closed quickly, but they're not the larger percentage of the patients ... There are really complex people frequently (CA Grp 6).

Nurses give similar accounts of dying patients being denied access to palliative care:

Eight years ago ... you could make the decision to bring somebody in. But now it's like I have to be very assertive with whoever is on call and say 'this patient's terminal. The family can't handle it. They need to come in for a terminal admit' ... and you have to get really in their face about it (CA Grp 6).

The policy around Do Not Resuscitate (DNR) orders was of notable concern to some California nurses. A DNR order, one nurse describes, 'goes on your file' and at least in her Managed Care organisation, 'stays there. ... It doesn't go away at the end of that hospitalization; ... you [are] in that status until you die' (CA Grp 5). Such orders can encourage non-treatment, especially if high costs are involved. Take the case of:

> a really sweet lady. ... She had been sick like a year before, had been on a vent for a few weeks. It was a horrible experience and she had made it clear to her family she did not want to be ventilated again ... She got pneumonia ... They wanted to put her on the floor ... They said 'Well we don't want to keep her in ICU. We're not going to vent her. She's DNR'. ... What she needed was ... aggressive nursing care to take care of her lungs so she didn't have to go to vent or she didn't have to die ... the nurses fought to get her transferred, not to the floor but to a step down unit where she ... did get better and she's alive today. [The family] had no idea when they signed that 'don't do cardiac resuscitation', 'don't put her on a vent', the doctors thought it meant 'don't give her any care' (CA Grp 5).

While in this case it was the doctors who were denying the care, the nurses see doctors as being pressured by Managed Care policies to take this path. Indeed some nurses argue that the DNR status is:

> an economic strategy that ... [Managed Care] is pushing and expanding on a daily basis (CA Grp 5).

It is interesting to compare these accounts with those of B.C. nurses who do not report pressure to act on DNR orders, or as they refer to them, 'advanced directives'. As one nurse explained:

> Rather than have it tattooed on the back of your throat, 'Do Not Intubate', ... people have the right to change their mind (BC Grp 1).

Indeed, in B.C. nurses tell of many cases where, often on the family's insistence, they continue to treat in futile situations:

> We sent out a fellow ... who was a Degree Two which means no CPR, comfort measures [only] ... When he went [to the hospital], he was uncomfortable, he was in renal failure ... they called the family in and the doctor tried to talk to the family about his age and the fact that they had signed a Degree Two ... the niece apparently looked up at the doctor and said, 'Well, what are you saying? That you're not going to bother treating him because we signed that?' And he spent about a month in ICU and ... he died a very terrible death (BC Grp 3).

In sum, nurses from California argue that instead of providing better access to a wide range of services – acute, preventive and chronic – through a single entry point, Managed Care as a form of implicit rationing does the opposite. It uses the single entry point to prevent access to the entire range of services.

They have just been managing access to care, they haven't been managing the care (CA Grp 7).

Managed Care becomes, as one nurse described: 'Managed Denial' (CA Grp 4). Others have argued similarly that Managed Care connotes a denial of services and a fundamental dedication to profit (Cassell 1998). In response to this denial, patients often turn to emergency rooms where some assessment is guaranteed by law. The law itself, however, was a response to mounting evidence that many patients were denied care and many seek this care only when their conditions have reached the crisis stage.

The importance of costs and coverage is particularly illuminating in the case of resuscitative efforts. Unlike what Timmermans (1999) found of the decisions to ration lifesaving efforts in the U.S., California nurses' accounts do not reflect the influence of presumed social worth on these decisions. Instead, it seemed that insurance coverage was the most influential deciding factor. This is in contrast to the situation B.C. nurses face.

In B.C., access to most forms of care[5] is not based on ability to pay and cannot be denied but, one could argue, is delayed, based on the assessment of need. Such delays are undoubtedly increasing in light of the reorganisation (and in most cases, reduction) of services, but concerns about rationing through increased wait times was not a prominent feature of these nurses' accounts. This is perhaps because of its relative lack of salience in the everyday work of nurses as compared with the work of other health care providers, such as physicians. Moreover, there is also some indication in the nurses' accounts of democratic decision making in the cutting of duplication in B.C. Neither democratic decision-making nor regional co-ordination seem to happen in California and perhaps because of this was not even mentioned by the nurses there.

It should also be noted that waiting is not only an issue for patients in B.C.; nurses in California also tell of the excessive waiting times for patients – either through HMO call centres, in public clinics or in ERs – only to be later denied care. This is consistent with what others have found of care in the U.S. (Taft and Steward 2000). Similar to the concerns expressed by nurses in this study, Hancock (1993), who writes from a British nursing perspective, argues that queues and waiting for treatment – an implicit form of rationing – is causing problems because acute illness left untreated gives rise to further medical problems which serve to increase the overall costs of treatment and care. This represents yet another challenge to the claim of cost-effectiveness under Managed Care and, indeed, is an important criticism of waiting times in the Canadian health care system (*c.f.* Globerman 1991).

Another salient difference highlighted between California and B.C. was regarding the focus of preventive care and health promotion. In brief, preventive measures in California were much more disease-oriented and were not immune to the overall denial of care occurring there, whereas in B.C. measures tended to have a broader wellness orientation and have not been cut back to the extent that they have in California. One needs to exercise caution, however, in reading such a finding because as many have argued, the move toward health promotion in Canada can be used as a rationale for the reducing of medical services for the sick (Armstrong and Armstrong 1996, Light 1999).

Thus, it is with respect to the rationing of the *access* to various forms of care – acute, preventive, palliative – that the primary difference in California and B.C. nurses' experiences is revealed. As we turn to discuss strategies that implicitly ration the *amount* of care, we see greater similarities in the account of nurses in California and B.C.

Rationing amount of care: get patients out quickly

> If you do hospitalise them, get them out as quickly as possible and have them see as few specialists and providers and do as few procedures as possible (CA Grp 5).

Not only has access to care been managed, particularly in the U.S., the amount of care a patient receives once care is accessed, has also been managed. We first examine nurses' experiences with care pathways and then discuss the related issue of early discharge policies and increased patient-to-nurse ratios.

Care pathways
Care pathways are a type of clinical protocol used primarily in nursing (Mykhalovskiy, forthcoming; Timmermans and Berg 1997). They set out a series of multidisciplinary interventions to be carried out for a group of defined patients over a standard period of time. Despite their promise to facilitate the co-ordination of patient care, nurses in California tell of how care pathways *determine* decision-making and become another strategy to ration care. For example, one nurse detailed how 'there are only certain diagnoses [doctors are] allowed to admit on' (CA Grp 4). So instead of allowing the admission decision to be based on the particularities of the case and of the doctor's opinion, formulas are applied. The same kind of formulas are also used to determine length of stay, surgery, discharge and homecare visits, areas where nurses have had some professional discretion in the past. As another nurse detailed:

> A person comes in ... presenting certain symptoms of stroke on day one ... by day three the social worker is asking ... which nursing home are you going to be going to by day five, because they're looking for you to be out of the hospital (CA Grp 3).

Nurses' concerns about the severe restrictions on autonomy are not based primarily on professional self-interest; their objections are related more to the real problems they see as a result of the lack of flexibility in these rules and how they ignore individual conditions and circumstances. As one nurse put it:

> You may have a diabetic who comes in and you're supposed to do this and this and this. And this only works for that piece of paper. It doesn't work for that person [be]cause that person may have other complications ... But the determination of how that patient gets treated is based on that piece of paper, not on the patient (CA Grp 5).

An additional concern California nurses have with care pathways is their relationship to variations in the coverage of services by patients' insurers. In many cases, major treatment is 'supposed to be okayed by the insurance company'. Decisions about what is considered 'appropriate' care are thus made by the company rather than by the doctor or nurse. Several nurses in California told story after story about the amount of time devoted to negotiating with the insurance system on behalf of their patients:

> We investigate what their coverage is because we have to work with them and try and fill their needs ... we do fight a lot with insurers and try to negotiate [with] them ... it's really complicated ... They'll say, 'This part, Medicare should cover' 'No, MediCal should cover it' 'No, then insurance should cover it'. And so there are those kinds of things that we get to do a lot. And it does slow down the work and delays our clients (CA Grp 7).

Time spent negotiating coverage is time not spent providing care – another means by which implicitly to ration nursing care.

> I think that's a real way that the HMOs are really restricting care because they make it so difficult ... to get approval ... I feel like I'm spending a lot of my nursing time pushing insurance companies (CA Grp 7).

Too often, the nurses say, all this time is completely wasted because care is denied.

Nurses in B.C. have no accounts of time spent unravelling the web of health care coverage that the California nurses give because everyone in B.C., as in the rest of Canada, receives uniform coverage. However, B.C. nurses do tell of the increasing use of care pathways in their places of work. By way of contrast, their perspective is, for the most part, positive. For example, one nurse said they like knowing what they could and could not do, and this prevented them from having to chase down a doctor to sign off on various procedures or tests. This more positive perspective on care pathways may be due largely to the fact that they are still new in B.C. and are guidelines more than they are an implicit rationing tool that *must* be followed. When, however, the use of care pathways resulted in a move toward early discharge, B.C. nurses expressed similar concerns to those of the California nurses.

Early discharge

> When your hospital stay is not revenue producing anymore, suddenly your condition improves drastically and you're out the door. ... *treated and streeted* (CA Grp 9).

Part and parcel of care pathways as a method of rationing care are early discharge policies. The drive to save costs drives patients out of the hospital quickly and, because they have left too soon, back in again. As one California nurse described:

> [Length of stay] has been shortened so the 'criticalness' of the patient is accelerating because they're being bumped out of critical care, the intensive care unit, faster into a step-down unit, ... to a rehab place or home. And often times they haven't had the education and the time to truly heal. And so they have problems with either readmission or people who were discharged prematurely from intensive care to a step-down unit only to have a crisis ... with compounded complications (CA Grp 4).

Surgery, even of the complex kind, does not guarantee a hospital stay. Several nurses, for example, pointed out that the new practice was to send the 'mastectomy patients home post-op day one'. Early discharge seems to be the policy, whatever the patient's condition. The rationing of care resulting from reduced length of stay in hospital often shifts the burden of care to the individual or his/her family:

> What you'd see are people that are at home with very complex medication, not fully understanding the treatments with wounds that are still in need of care. ... More and more burden was shifted onto the family that necessarily doesn't have the skill to provide that care (CA Grp 4).

> We're sending a woman home with drains [after a mastectomy] to be cared for by her 80-year-old husband who's half blind and has had a stroke. That's home care (CA Grp 5).

B.C. nurses express similar concerns with early discharge policies:

> We also see patients coming out of hospital so much faster. The acuity of the patients is remarkable and the biggest thing I can think of is the

fact that people come out post mastectomy 24 hours post op. They come out and they've got a row of staples and maybe two drains that they are supposed to be able to manage and of course they can't (BC Grp 6).

and the need to teach patients more in less time:

A lot of the wards send patients home and they haven't taught them a thing because they haven't had time ... Give them a syringe and say poke it in your leg, you know. Home care may be there in two days. If you feel weird, phone your doctor (BC Grp 1).

Nurses in B.C. also tell of increased recidivism resulting from increasing implementation of early discharge policies:

I've certainly heard ... 'You guys are sending them home too early and we're getting them back' (BC Grp 1).

With respect to home care, nurses in B.C. tell of still having more discretion than that of which California nurses speak. As one B.C. nurse states:

I've had days when I've said, 'You know, this person is going to take me three hours to do. Don't give me more than three patients. I can't do any more'. And everybody says, 'Fine' (BC Grp 2).

But these choices are disappearing, or at least becoming more circumscribed as home care becomes increasingly rationed:

We used to put in ... a live-in, someone to come to stay with someone for 24 hours a day ... And if it took eight months, well, it took eight months. ... Now we're to the point where we have strict [limits]. ... So then your options are you pay privately (BC Grp 9).

This burden on home care has been exacerbated by the shift from institutional to community care, arguably an economic strategy that not only shifts care but also costs to the patient, given the lack of public provision for home care in B.C. and elsewhere in Canada (Armstrong & Armstrong 1998). These new 'maximums' in B.C. are 'old hat' in California – but they are not based on individual insurance coverage – *everyone* is reduced.

Dividing up care and increasing patient-to-nurse ratios

More patients, sicker patients, less help, less equipment. Less, less, less (CA Grp 9).

Another implicit method of rationing the amount of care includes increasing patient-to-nurse ratios, which in turn decreases the overall amount of nursing care each patient gets. This, in addition to the increased acuity of patients resulting from early discharge policies, results in much heavier workloads for nurses. Strategies to ensure that only the minimum number of nurses are on duty at any point in time cross cut California and B.C. As a nurse in B.C. states:

> When you get a crunch, *i.e.* ... they want to send you two more patients, you're supposed to get together in this little huddle ... and as a group make a decision as to who you think could handle another patient ... I mean, it's wonderful on paper, but it's not functional because you're all too busy to get together in this little huddle and have a discussion. And besides nobody wants another patient (BC Grp 1).

Another B.C. nurse points out that even though management claims, 'they haven't really cut' she replies:

> No [they] haven't cut but you need one hell of a lot more because for instance where I work, the open heart area, we kept them for two days in ICU before they ever came out on the ward, but now you're sending them out to the ward in less then 24 hours but you're not increasing the nursing staff (BC Grp 1).

A nurse in an intensive care unit in California similarly explained how her work load had intensified, leaving her with less time per patient:

> We had a nine-patient capacity unit ... that was when we were totally full. Rarely did we have nine patients. Five to seven was our average. Well now, with all the hospital closures, increase of severity of illness in patients and the lack of critical care beds, we've expanded this other ICU so now rather than be in charge of five to nine patients, last night I was in charge of 15 in two separate units. ... almost double your workload (CA Grp 9).

The speed-up means 'it's not possible to do physically' (CA Grp 5) what needs to be done, let alone what the nurses think should be done based on their training and experience. 'You're just doing tasks on them now' (CA Grp 3). There is no time left to provide the kind of quality care nurses see as both rewarding and necessary:

> Activities that used to be integral to our nursing practice are now becoming superfluous, as defined by management. ... What they've done is referred now to essential care ... so you're here to do essential care and they actually list the tasks that we're expected to do and all these other things that are nursing care are not essential (CA Grp 5).

One nurse called it 'nursing maintenance [because] it's not nursing anymore (CA Grp 9). But it is not just 'non-essential' nursing care that is not being done. In some cases, 'essential' nursing care is not being done:

> We had a real problem at my facility with patients becoming septic – they have arterial, central lines – and the reason they're becoming septic ... is because the dressings were supposed to be changed every second day on some lines, every third day on other lines, and the nurses are not doing it ... They're ignoring it because they've got to ignore something because they can't do the work (CA Grp 5).

A nurse in B.C. voiced similar concerns:

> I guess we just work harder ... [but] the nurses have not yet let the patients slide. We're injuring ourselves and burning out ... I hear the nurses ... say, 'We stay overtime now because we're not prepared to give up that care', and ... I don't mean just time talking. I mean time changing a dressing that really should be changed (BC Grp 1).

The implicit rationing of nursing care by increasing patient-to-nurse ratios is exacerbated by cuts to other ancillary personnel[6]. One nurse explained that in practice this means 'one day I literally lost my unit assistant, my house-keeper and was told they were decreasing my staffing' (CA Grp 9). Another California nurse told how:

> We're emptying ... our own garbage. We're emptying the linen. We're doing so much that it's almost impossible to give that holistic care to someone (CA Grp 5).

Nurses in B.C. reported similarly that 'We no longer have housecleaning, except for emergency' (BC Grp 7). Several nurses felt, 'that's why our infection rate is going up ... now that they've taken away all the house-keeping staff' (BC Grp 7).

In sum, it is in rationing the amount of nursing care – through care pathways, early discharge policies and reduced nurse staffing levels – where greater similarities between California and B.C. are revealed. In both cases, nurses' critiques are not dissimilar to Ritzer's (1996) 'McDonaldization' thesis. Care pathways and early discharge policies could be likened to the introduction of sameness and the principles of fast food production to nursing care: making people fit the product and making that product the same for all people.

The main impetus underlying these similarities can be linked directly to the flow of managerial policies from the U.S. to Canada. This is why we find that the changes that this entails for B.C. nurses have not come as far as they have in California or as fast. Just as Wells (1995: 738) has noted in the

U.K., 'recent changes to the organisational values in the NHS are leading to similar issues arising already faced by American nurses'. Specifically, the principles of equity, comprehensiveness, equality of access and free delivery of care traditionally associated with the British NHS, and with the Canadian health care system, are increasingly confronted by the organisation/management values of efficiency, effectiveness, quality, choice and satisfying the needs of the consumer.

The collision of these two different sets of values is particularly salient when comparing the accounts of nurses in California and B.C. regarding the bureaucratization of care in part through the differential implementation of care pathways. Similar to Hunter's (1997) argument that bureaucracy is a form of rationing, nurses in California reveal that much of their time is spent negotiating care with insurance companies and that both directly – in terms of denial of care – and indirectly – through time spent away from the bedside – rations care. That nurses in B.C. did not make mention of this is largely to do with the different health care system contexts these nurses are working in – one set of care pathways in B.C. depending on need because of one payer; several in California depending on insurance coverage.

In presenting nurses' critique of care pathways and early discharge policies, it is important to tease apart the focus on managerial policies, some of which are based on evidence, and EBP itself. It is not necessarily EBP that these nurses are wary of – indeed, nurses in B.C. spoke quite positively about its potential – but of its inconsistent translation into managerial policies. From these nurses' perspective, it seems that those EBPs that entail cost savings, such as early discharge, are readily implemented, whereas those that do not necessarily yield cost savings, such as broader health promotion measures, are not only not implemented, in the California setting where short-term profits seem to be of particular concern, they are increasingly being cut back. This is consistent with recent examinations of nurses' perceptions of barriers to EBP (Newman et al. 1998, Retsas 2000) which pointed to the lack of organisational support to use fully research in nursing care policies. This ambiguity towards EBP and its differential implementation is not unlike what has been found of physicians in Canada (Rappolt 1997) and other settings (c.f., Dent 1999, Mayer and Piterman 1999). Orentlicher (1998) similarly argues that practice guidelines are not necessarily objective, medically based measures but are heavily value-laden, and the value judgments that they inevitably make are camouflaged under a veneer of scientific objectivity.

Conclusions

In conclusion, the key differences that arise from this comparative analysis of nurses' views of rationing care concern the issue of rationing access to various forms of care; similarities are revealed in nurses' accounts of the rationing of the amount of that care. The differences in the experiences of rationing by nurses in California and B.C. we feel in large part can be traced back to the differences in the organisation of their respective health care systems – access to care being guaranteed in the Canadian system and not in the U.S. One could also argue that these differences may also be in part a reflection of the different occupational cultures of Canadian and U.S. nurses. If this were the case, however, we would be less likely to see the kind of similarities we found with respect to nurses' experiences with care pathways, early discharge policies and reduced staffing. Indeed, the similarities we found here are arguably due to the cross-border transfer of managerial policies. Thus, as we stated before, it is difficult to divorce the micro-experiences of health care providers from the broader context within which they are working.

Our research may seem to suggest that the debate on rationing or on the management of care in general is less well developed in Canada than in the U.S. But it is important to note that this may be due to the state and province that we chose as our referents for these two systems. Indeed, the rationing and managing of care is much more widespread in other Canadian provinces, such as Ontario, than it is in B.C. and perhaps less so in other states than it is in California. Hence, caution must be taken in over-generalising these findings beyond California and B.C. to broad U.S./ Canada differences. They do, however, give us some indication that the outcome of rationing through the management of health care, as experienced by nurses, may not be better care for more, as is claimed and as some nurses hope (Huey 1990), but poorer care to fewer people. Indeed, we find that from the perspective of nurses there is little evidence that Managed Care is working in the U.S. where it is deeply embedded, and therefore question how suitable a model it is for Canada and elsewhere where it is just beginning to be applied.

Acknowledgements

The authors were like to thank the editors, David Hughes and Donald Light, for the opportunity to contribute to this Monograph. We would also like to thank the two anonymous reviewers for their helpful and insightful comments on earlier drafts of this chapter. The research this chapter is based on was funded by the Social Sciences and Humanities Research Council of Canada through a Standard Research Grant.

Notes

1   We capitalise Managed Care to refer to a specific set of practices around the management of care adopted from the private sector.

2   Even government programmes like Medicare and Medicaid have shifted their beneficiaries to private Managed Care plans primarily to save money (McMillan 1993).
3   Callahan (1998) argues that it is not a stated goal of Managed Care to achieve universal care; indeed, there are strong financial incentives in Managed Care *not* to enroll an unlimited number of people indiscriminately.
4   Those who insist on their right to an annual pap smear may continue to have one. The consequence is a two-tier system within the Managed Care programme, with the least educated going without the preventative care while others may get more than they need.
5   One exception to this is home care which is not universally covered under government health care.
6   The greater cuts among non-RNs in California are partly explained by Title 22, a state regulation which sets the minimum number of RNs required – one nurse for every two patients in intensive care or for high RN levels in other units. So a minimum number of RNs, at least in theory, must be maintained, whatever the classification system or management says. There is no equivalent legislation, however, for ancillary workers.

References

Andrews, J. (1993) Rational rationing, *Nursing Standard*, 17, 37, 22–3.

Armstrong, P. and Armstrong, H. (1996) *Wasting Away: the Undermining of Canadian Health Care*. Toronto: Oxford University Press.

Armstrong, P. and Armstrong, H. (1998) *Universal Health Care: What the United States Can Learn from the Canadian Experience*. New York: New Press.

Baines, D.L., Tolley, K. and Whynes, D.K. (1998) The ethics of resource allocation: the views of general practitioners in Lincolnshire, U.K., *Social Science and Medicine*, 47, 1555–64.

Blake, D.C. (1994) Should medical care be a right without restrictions by cost, age, citizenship, prognosis, or self-infliction, *Activities, Adaptation and Aging*, 18, 107–21.

Bloomfield, B.P. (1991) The role of information systems in the UK National Health Service: action at a distance and the fetish of calculation, *Social Studies of Science*, 212, 701–34.

Callahan, D. (1998) Managed care and the goals of medicine, *Journal of the American Geriatrics Society*, 46, 385–8.

Carrasquillo, O., Himmelstein, D.U., Woolhandler, S. and Bor, D.H. (1999) Trends in health insurance coverage, 1989–1997, *International Journal of Health Services*, 29, 467–83.

Cassell, E.J. (1998) The future of the doctor-payer-patient relationship, *Journal of the American Geriatric Society*, 46, 318–21.

Conrad, P. and Brown, P. (1993) Rationing medical care: a sociological reflection, *Research in the Sociology of Health Care*, 10, 3–22.

Coombs, B. (1990) Two ethics compete in debate on health care rationing, *Journal of the American Academy of Physician Assistants*, 3, 436–9.

Daniels, N. (1985) *Just Health Care*. New York: Cambridge University Press.

Daniels, N. (1986) Why saying no to patients in the United States is so hard – cost containment, justice and provider autonomy, *New England Journal of Medicine*, 314, 1380–3.

Daniels, N., Light, D. and Caplan, R. (1986) *Benchmarks of Fairness for Health Care Reform*. New York: Oxford University Press.

Davis, A.J. (1991) The allocation of health care resources, *Ethical Issues in Nursing Research*, 13, 136–7.

Dent, M.P. (1999) Professional judgement and the role of clinical guidelines and EBM: Netherlands, Britain and Sweden, *Journal of Interprofessional Care*, 13, 151–64.

Goold, S. (1996) Allocating health care: cost-utility analysis, informed democratic decision making, or the veil of ignorance? *Journal of Health Politics, Policy and Law*, 2, 69–98.

Globerman, S. (1991) Hospital waiting lists in B.C.: evidence and policy implications, *Policy Studies Review*, 10, 45–60.

Grimshaw, J.M. and Hutchinson, A. (1995) Clinical practice guidelines – do they enhance value for money in health care? *British Medical Bulletin*, 51, 927–40.

Hancock, C. (1993) Getting a quart out of a pint pot. In British Medical Association (ed), *Rationing in Action*. London: British Medical Journal Publishing Group.

Huey, F. (1990) Rationing rationing, *Geriatric Nursing: American Journal of Care for the Aging*, 11, 215.

Hughes, D. and Griffiths, L. (1996) 'But if you look at the coronary anatomy...'. risk and rationing in cardiac surgery, *Sociology of Health and Illness*, 18, 172–97.

Hughes, D. and Griffiths, L. (1997) 'Ruling in' and 'ruling out': two approaches to the micro-rationing of health care, *Social Science and Medicine*, 44, 589–99.

Hunter, D.J. (1997) *Desperately Seeking Solutions: Rationing Health Care*. New York: Longman.

Klein, R., Day, P. and Redmayne, S. (1996) *Managing Scarcity: Priority Setting and Rationing in the National Health Service*. Buckingham: Open University Press.

Light, D. (1999) *The Real Ethics of Rationing Upstream: Is the Canadian Government Putting Patients Last?* The 1998 John F. McCreary Lecture. Vancouver: University of British Columbia.

Mariner, W.K. (1995) Rationing health care and the need for credible scarcity: why Americans can't say no, *American Journal of Public Health*, 85, 1439–45.

Mayer, J. and Piterman, L. (1999) The attitudes of Australian GPs to evidence-based medicine: a focus group study, *Family Practice*, 16, 627–32.

McMillan, A. (1993) Trends in Medicare health maintenance organization enrollment: 1986–93, *Health Care Financing Review*, 15, 135–46.

Mittelstadt, P. (1985) The future of our nation's health care: will rationing be needed? *American Journal of Occupational Therapy*, 39, 229–32.

Mykhalovskiy, E. (forthcoming) Troubled hearts, care pathways and hospital restructuring: exploring health services research as active knowledge, *Studies in Cultures, Organizations, and Societies*.

Newman, M., Papadoupoulos, I. and Sigsworth, J. (1998) Barriers to evidence-based practice, *Intensive and Critical Care Nursing*, 14, 231–8.

Orentlicher, D. (1998) Practice guidelines: a limited role in resolving rationing decisions, *Journal of the American Geriatric Society*, 46, 369–72.

Perrin, K. (1989) Rationing health care: should it be done? *Journal of Gerontological Nursing*, 15, 10–14.

Rappolt, S. (1997) Clinical guidelines and the fate of medical autonomy in Ontario, *Social Science and Medicine*, 44, 977–87.

Reigle, J. (1990) Resource allocation decisions in critical care nursing, *Nursing Clinics of North America*, 24, 1009–15.

Retsas, A. (2000) Barriers to using research evidence in nursing practice, *Journal of Advanced Nursing*, 31, 599–606.

Ritzer, G. (1996) *The McDonaldization of Society*. Thousand Oaks, Ca: Pine Forge Press.

Stevens, P.E. (1992) Who gets care? Access to health care as an arena for nursing action, *Scholarly Inquiry for Nursing Practice*, 6, 185–200.

Taft, K. and Steward, G. (2000) *Clear Answers: the Economic and Politics of For-Profit Medicine*. Edmonton, Alberta: University of Alberta Press.

Timmermans, S. and Berg, M. (1997) Standardization in action: achieving local universality through medical protocols, *Social Studies of Science*, 27, 273–305.

Timmermans, S. (1999) When death isn't dead: implicit social rationing during resuscitative efforts, *Sociological Inquiry*, 69, 51–75.

Tuohy, C.J. (1999) *Accidental Logics: The Dynamics of Change in the Health Care Arena in the United States, Britain and Canada*. New York: Oxford University Press.

Ubel, P.A. and Goold, S. (1997) Recognizing bedside rationing: clear cases and tough calls, *Annals of Internal Medicine*, 126, 74–80.

Wells, J.S.G. (1995) Health care rationing: nursing perspectives, *Journal of Advanced Nursing*, 22, 738–44.

6

Rationing health care to disabled people

Gary L. Albrecht

Introduction

The rationing of health care to disabled people is one of the most persistent and perplexing problems facing contemporary societies regardless of their geographical location, political orientation, cultural values or level of economic development. Much attention has been given to how emphasis on the 'rugged individual' and the forces of capitalism have played out in the United States health arena through managed care organisations and rationing mechanisms (Light 2000). The conjoint effect of these corporate and institutional forces has been to compromise fairness where insurance companies 'charge more or pay less than actuarially fair risk rating would justify' (Light 1992: 2503, Stone 1993), insure that much of the health care system is driven by profit motives (Albrecht 1992), and accept that governments do not provide an adequate safety net for vulnerable populations (Stone 1988). Disabled people are at particular risk of rationing because they are often disqualified from insurance programmes because of 'pre-existing conditions', or are judged not to be 'good' financial or social investments. The result is that disabled people frequently do not receive the care they need, the care is disjointed, not delivered in a timely fashion, it is reactive rather than preventive, and the care system is not transparent to the consumer (Albrecht and Bury 2001).

While the scholarly commentary on managed care and rationing of services to disabled people focuses mainly on the United States, similar institutional dynamics are playing out in many other countries. It cannot be assumed that 'different' social values, a more community-oriented culture, stronger family structures, or existing social welfare systems will protect disabled people outside the US from the influence of managed care and rationing forces. Growing demands on the health care, disability and rehabilitation infrastructures are global phenomena that affect governments in many nations. The largest and most powerful health care, managed care, insurance, pharmaceutical and medical supply corporations are international in organisation, global in reach and market driven (Albrecht and Bury 2001). For example, as early as 1984, Robert Evans (1984) pointed to the mounting equity problems and rationing issues present in the Canadian health care system. Light (1995), Griffiths and Hughes (1998) and Hughes *et al.* (1997) have insightfully analysed how health markets have formed and evolved in Britain with complex forms of implicit and explicit rationing becoming increasingly apparent. Brudevold *et al.* (2000) indicate how managed care concepts and rationing are occurring in Hong Kong and seem to be applied throughout Asia. The same story is true in Latin America where international managed care companies like Aetna, EXXEL and Cigna have moved into Latin health marketplaces in joint ventures with companies in Mexico, Brazil, Argentina and Chile, applying American marketplace strategies including the rationing of care (Stocker *et al.* 1999). The problems and dynamics of the marketplace and the rationing of care remain similar in these numerous nations but are expressed somewhat differently according to culture, context and resources. Since the detailed analysis of these forces across many countries is beyond the scope of this chapter, I will concentrate on how managed care and the rationing of care impact on disabled people in the United States, realising that there might also be important applications to other countries and settings.

This chapter uses a political economic perspective to inform the analysis: How does the system work and whom does it benefit? While other political economic analyses of disability address the societal level (Albrecht 1992), this chapter concentrates on the micro level of how medical care in a managed care environment is experienced by disabled consumers. The analysis identifies the major stakeholders and the political economic forces that influence individual, family and organisational decision making. The disparity between the concept of managed care and the experienced reality will be examined. Finally, the consequences of rationing care for disabled people are explored.

The contentiousness of disability definitions and models

Any discussion of disability in today's scholarly and political arenas is fraught with controversy over definitions, models, ideology and purpose. The debates essentially focus on what disability is, where it resides, what it means, who controls its definition, how society constructs it, how it is experienced, who is responsible for it and what are its consequences. Polar disagreements have focused on the differences between the medical and social models of disability. These often reduce complex arguments and realities to an emphasis on the organic, individual, medical treatment and power over the 'patient' versus an emphasis on the environment and the larger 'disabling society' that shapes disability through its definitional and social control mechanisms (Llewellyn and Hogan 2000, Hedlund 2000).

Arguments over concepts, ideologies, measurement instruments and a wide range of purposes of disability definitions often revolve around debate over the ICIDH, the Global Burden of Disease project, the perceived value of life and social welfare policies (Albrecht and Verbrugge 2000, Pfeiffer 2000, Bury 2000a, Altman 2001, Williams 2001).

Because of these ongoing debates, no agreed definition of disability exists in the literature. For the purposes of this study, disability is conceptualised as having an organic component (related to impairment) but as being primarily constituted through the interaction of individuals with their 'bodies', social contexts and larger society. Disabled peoples' social interactions with others, and their roles, are limited by the physical and social environment which influences their self identities, their power over their circumstances, their responsibility for actions and their place in society. The two cases analysed in this chapter are grounded in all these aspects of the disability reality and experience.

Negotiating health care for the chronically ill

Charmaz (1991), Strauss (1993), Thorne (1993) and Seymour (1998) have provided insightful analyses of what it means to live with a chronic illness, deal with the health care system, remake the body and re-establish an identity for people with chronic illnesses, in three different countries. The first two are classic interactionist studies which examine how chronically ill people interpret their experiences and reconstruct their lives, identities, body and social relationships through interaction with others over time. Strauss also details how the chronically ill negotiate with the powerful medical establishment and larger society to re-constitute their places in the social order. Thorne's Canadian study is closer to the present research because it moves on from an account of the chronic illness experience to chart some of 'the flaws in modern health care organisation and ideology' (1993: x). She describes the experiences of the chronically ill, providing poignant detail on how they negotiate their care and develop strategies to deal with the powerful health care providers in an institutional context. She emphasises the difficulty of establishing a trusting relationship with care providers and with the debilitating force of institutional authority. On the organisational level, she describes and analyses how the chronically ill struggle with professional power and incompetence, 'falling through the cracks', dehumanising experiences, health care politics and bureaucracy and being caught in endless 'red tape'. In an Australian study, Seymour (1998) adds to this discourse by analysing how being 'embodied' increases understanding of what it is like for disabled people physically and socially to remake an impaired body. As an illustration she suggests that the process of reconstructing the self is interwoven with social expectations which require continual interaction and adjustment for everyone involved in the process.

These studies inform the present work but this study differs from them in three important ways. First, three of the four studies discussed above focus on chronically ill not disabled people. Chronic illness concentrates on the personal, the subjective experience of illness which in conjunction with an impairment may or may not result in a disability. Second, these studies were conducted at a time or in a context where the inexorable forces of managed care and rationing of care were not as apparent, forceful or as disruptive as today, particularly in the American setting. Third, these studies used symbolic interaction, negotiation and embodiment theories to analyse behaviour on the individual level and in the interactions between the individual, professionals and care organisations. The present study differs from them in that it examines how macro level, political economic forces impinge on disabled people on the micro level to change or intensify the nature of their experiences and negotiations in the health care arena.

The political economy of disability

Political economists have developed theories to address two fundamental, inter-related questions: '(1) How do institutions evolve in response to individual incentives, strategies, and choices? And, (2) How do institutions affect the performance of political and economic systems?' (Alt and Alesina 1996: 645). In the disability context, political economic analysts investigated how institutions act to structure and control the marketplace, develop products and stimulate demand (Albrecht and Bury 2001). This political economic work on the institutional level has corollaries on the micro level. From the perspective of disabled people and their families, two questions persist: (1) How and with what effect do disabled people express their needs and desires in the health care marketplace? and, (2) what is their experience with the subsequent institutional responses to their health problems and desire to live independently?

I have earlier examined historically (Albrecht 1992) how rehabilitation goods and services were transformed into commodities in Western capitalist nations in response to defining disability as a social problem. In this disability business, "consumers, providers, investors, and regulators profit and/ or lose in the transactions" (Albrecht 1992: 27). This is in stark contrast to earlier traditions of caring for disabled people in families, communities and charitable institutions where profit was not of primary concern in the health and welfare sector (Castel 1995). I analysed stakeholder groups in terms of their relative power and mutual interdependency. These groups included hospitals, insurance companies, pharmaceutical corporations, medical supply and technology industries, health care professionals, therapy businesses and home care agencies, law practices, banks and accounting firms specialising in disability, government and lobby groups, politicians and finally the consumer. As expected, the least powerful group was the disabled consumers who, although being the most vulnerable, created the demand for the entire system to prosper. To provide perspective on the operation and outcomes of such national disability systems, it is essential to examine the disability business from the perspectives of disabled consumers and their families (Rier 2000).

Rationing medical care to disabled people

Since administrative decision makers, policy makers and even the tax paying public recognise that demand for rehabilitation and disability-related services can potentially be unlimited and the system abused, rationing of care is imperative (Jensen *et al.* 1997). From the corporate managers' and policy makers' vantagepoint, a strong demand for disability goods and services is necessary for the disability business to thrive. If demand is not kept under control, however, increased system access and escalating costs can threaten corporate profits or place an unbearable burden on government budgets.

The institutional response to these pressures has been a rationing of disability goods and services through social policies and managerial decisions employed to allocate scarce resources according to implicit or explicit criteria. Explicit rationing occurs when governments and/or insurance groups apply formal criteria to disabled people, defining which conditions, treatments and services will be covered and how much access to care will be allowed. Such a system is difficult to operationalise because of the complexity in disabling conditions and variability in required care over time for similar conditions (Mechanic 1995, Charmaz 2000). Implicit rationing occurs when a third party, such as a physician or manager employed by a Health Maintenance Organisation (HMO), National Health Service (NHS) or other managed care organisation, negotiates the type and amount of care to be delivered with the consumer within the confines of a general set of organisational rules and market forces. Both the explicit and implicit criteria publicly focus on the perceived need (medical necessity) of disabled people but often encompass other variables such as amount of available resources, cost of treatment, the likely outcome of the intervention, competing demands made on limited resources, public support for disability programmes, social values, ethical considerations and the economic and political profit potential for the institutional stakeholders involved (Harrison and Moran 2000). In the case of implicit rationing, the consumer is at a considerable disadvantage in negotiation because the power relationship and information networks are asymmetrical in favour of the providing professionals or institutions.

In developed countries such as the United Kingdom, the United States, Germany and New Zealand, attempts were initially made to control disability costs by rationing care at the supply side, but when these efforts were judged to have limited success, attention was turned to managing demand for access to care, goods and services (Garvey 1993). These countries employed a third-party payment system to limit demand through implicit rationing, where the act of paying for disability care was detached from the disabled person requiring that care. The theory is that a neutral third party will be able to make more objective decisions about medical necessity, likely outcome and effective use of limited resources than the self-interested consumer or purchaser of the goods and services.

In principle, this makes sense but does not take the political and financial interests of the third party into account (Iezoni 1999). In many industrial countries, a multitude of third-party systems exist which divide their work usually according to the risk characteristics of the populations served (Bodenheimer and Casalino 1999). The poorer, disabled people are most often found in different insurance risk pools and delivery systems, with more limited resources than the richer, healthier people (Luft and Miller 1988, Hornbrook and Goodman 1996, Banja and DeJong 2000). As a consequence, disabled people are unlikely to receive the same level of benefits and are treated differently from wealthier, healthier citizens, thus creating a fundamental social inequity (Mehlman *et al.* 1997, Dudley *et al.* 1998, Druss *et al.* 2000). From a political economic perspective, such systems work well for the privileged until they or members of their families become disabled (Harris *et al.* 2000). Let us now turn our attention to the way in which the third-party payers, the managed care systems, ration care to disabled people, and address what the outcomes and consequences are for them and the larger society.

Methods

This study is based on an in-depth, longitudinal analysis of two cases that were identified and followed as part of a larger ethnographic/interview study of 153 disabled people living in the community. The larger study, conducted from September 1996 to December 1999 in the Chicago metropolitan area, used focus groups, ethnographic methods and semi-structured interviews with disabled people in their homes and community settings to ascertain how they lived their daily lives. Particular attention was given to how disabled people defined their social worlds, adapted to their environments, established social networks, discovered and accessed sources of health and medical care, dealt with the 'grinding problems' of everyday life, and how they attempted to enhance the quality of their lives. The common bond among these people was the disability experience. Some of them had reliable access to medical care and social services, but most struggled to have their problems recognised and dealt with in an integrated and timely fashion. The detailed methods of the larger study are described elsewhere (Albrecht and Devlieger 1999: 977–88).

As the larger study was being completed, it became apparent that most disabled people experienced significant difficulties in dealing with managed care organisations and various rationing mechanisms operating in both the public and private sectors. Frequently this was expressed as a lack of access to appropriate care, a lack of continuity and integration of care, uncertainty and stress and continual worries about paying for care. The emotional and financial burdens of continually battling with the health care system exacerbated the problems of living with a disability. The investigator decided that these issues deserved an in-depth examination on the micro level to understand the experience and dynamics of rationed care for disabled people. After a review of the focus group notes, ethnographic materials and interview notes from the larger study, the investigator selected two cases, representative of individuals in the larger group, based on the study participants' disabilities, personal characteristics, previous medical history, insurance status, education, supportive family, living arrangements, problematic experiences with managed and rationed care and willingness to participate in this related but extended study.

The two participants represented two major types of disability. One had a physical disability resulting from a post-polio condition; the other experienced disability related to chronic depression. These two individuals were the 'good news' stories of the disability world because they were not in that group in the United Stakes that had fallen through the safety net and they did have considerable resources to deal with their problems. These two individuals were closely followed from 1 January 1997 to 31 December 1999.

One of the individuals was a 49-year-old, married white female primary school teacher, with grown-up children, who belonged to a Preferred Provider Organisation (PPO) type of managed care insurance plan offered through work. 'Sylvia' (both names are pseudonyms) had experienced chronic depression over a period of eight years with intermittent serious episodes brought on by stressful life events. She was medically diagnosed with unipolar major depression, treated with antidepressants and psychiatric therapy and had been hospitalised for one week in 1997 for her condition. This disability periodically prevented her from going to work, cooking, housekeeping and engaging in routine social activities. During her bouts of depression, she felt flat affect, had little energy and would often stay in bed to rest and sleep for long periods of time. She was fortunate because she had a supportive family and friends, adequate health insurance and an understanding employer during this period.

This is a good example of a chronic disabling mental condition because unipolar major depression is formally recognised by the DSM IV diagnostic manual, deemed treatable – though not curable – by mental health clinicians, is presently estimated to be the number four cause of disability world-wide and projected to be the number two cause by 2020 (Murray and Lopez 1996). In the United States, major depression is the leading cause of disability but in 1997 only 23 per cent of adults diagnosed with the condition received treatment (Centers for Disease Control 2000). This is due in part to the refusal of many managed care groups to permit the treatment of 'pre-existing medical conditions' and the public expectation that they will act in this way (Scheier 2000).

The second individual was a 48-year-old married white male with grown-up children and a college education who worked as a project manager in a research institution, had had polio at the age of four and since that event had experienced post-polio syndrome. 'Steve' has been using a wheelchair, a modified van and work environment, and modifications in his home, as well as having a personal care assistant (PA), to be able to live independently. He had Blue Cross/Blue Shield insurance from California that he had transported with him when he moved to his present position. Technically, he is on disability retirement from the Los Angeles School system, but is permitted to earn a modest income to supplement his disability retirement benefits. His medical care is operated under a managed care model. He is fortunate in having above-average insurance, a supportive wife and son, and a reasonably accommodating environment that allows independent living. Post-polio syndrome is a good example of a chronic physically disabling condition because it is readily diagnosed, clearly visible due to wheelchair use, generally does not involve cognitive nor communicative difficulties and is relatively unstigmatised (partly because of the positive image of famous 'sufferers' such as President Franklin Delano Roosevelt).

The purpose of the study and the methods were explained to the two disabled subjects and their spouses and they agreed to participate. A combination of ethnographic, semi-structured interview and diary methods were employed, together with selective interviews with some providers and managed care decision makers related to their cases who were interviewed in person or on the telephone by the investigator. During the course of the study both disabled participants experienced a critical medical event that unravelled over time requiring them to seek care for an acute episode of a chronic condition. In each case they were evaluated, treated and followed up at home. The study participants were encouraged to keep a diary of their disability-related problems and contacts with health care and social service providers. They were encouraged to record what happened and, when problems arose, to ask the pertinent health care/stakeholder representatives what they did and why they did it. In addition, both couples had extensive medical, insurance and financial records. These activities and records were essential in helping the couples exercise some control over their own treatment. Both couples were interviewed four times at length in their homes or in the community during the three years of the study and extensive ethnographic notes were taken. Additionally single interviews were conducted with two physicians and three managed care decisions makers who had had dealings with the main subjects.

All of the interviews were recorded in writing as the participants and providers declined to be tape recorded. The ethnographic, interview and diary data were content analysed for critical events in the unfolding story, temporal sequence, dominant themes, participant assessment of environmental forces at work, announced rationale of the actors' actions and for some of the after-the-fact explanations. Since the case study was longitudinal, the participants were interviewed in succeeding cycles about some of the ambiguities in the data and about their interpretations of what had transpired. Furthermore, the participants were encouraged to ask providers and managed care representatives about what had happened and about the rationale for the actions when these were not clear. Again, these data were content analysed. After the investigator had identified critical events and analysed the explanations of what had occurred, he checked out these facts and interpretations with the study participants. This strategy thus employed a form of participatory action research method where the disabled people and their spouses performed an active role in the problem definition, gathering of evidence and interpretation of results.

These two cases are important because arguably they are representative of a substantial group of disabled people in the larger study who had problematic dealings with managed care organisations and the rationing of care. This addresses the issue of external validity in the case study. The two case studies are prospective, capture structural forces and processes operating over time, use multiple methods and sources of data to triangulate on the issues. Furthermore, they provide a 'thick description' of these disability care-management dynamics, attempt to grasp the multiple interpretations of events and actions of the major stakeholders in the activity, and use the principles of participatory action research in case studies (Stake 2000, Miller and Crabtree 2000). Such a design addresses major issues concerning internal validity (Handwerker and Borgatti 1998).

Results

Case one

The critical event studied in Sylvia's case occurred in the Autumn of 1998 when she experienced a bout of severe depression which was exacerbated by her medical intolerance to Zoloft and Prozac prescribed by her psychiatrist in the hope of controlling the symptoms. Her depression was occasioned by a series of conflictful interchanges with her ageing mother who continually criticised her decisions, her values, the rearing of her children, spoke ill of her to her children and told her repeatedly that she did not love her. Her mother was reported as saying, 'You know that I always wished that you had been a boy'. As Sylvia fell deeper into depression and was unable to carry out the activities of her daily life, her husband suggested, and she agreed, that she revisit her psychiatrist for help. She told both her husband and her psychiatrist, 'I can't go on like this'. Because of her previous medical history, serious reactions to the anti-depressants, and becoming even more depressed during the initial sessions of therapy, her psychiatrist suggested electro-convulsive therapy (ECT) which she said was often effective with severe chronic depression. Sylvia was reluctant because she had heard of many popular 'horror stories' about this treatment and she knew that it was very invasive, with side effects like temporary loss of memory and nausea. She was desperate but fearful: 'I know I've got to do something but I'm afraid'. She did know of a close friend who had been similarly depressed, had unsuccessfully tried every conceivable remedy but ultimately tried a course of ECT which worked marvels for her. Her friend told her, 'If it worked for me, it might be the answer for you'.

Given the seriousness of the situation, Sylvia and her husband decided to research ECT, look for alternatives and talk to others who had had the treatment. But this had to be done in a hurry because the condition was worsening. After consulting a number of psychiatrists, talking with others who had had similar experiences and reading a number of recommended articles (Janicak *et al.* 1997, Eist 1998, Fink 1999), her choices narrowed to intensive psychotherapy, starting a new antidepressant, taking a course of ECT, trying an experimental treatment of Repetitive Transcranial Magnetic Stimulation (rTMS) or doing nothing (Beedle *et al.* 1998). Sylvia felt acute distress so she wanted to do something immediately, but did not want to undertake a course of intensive psychotherapy and had already had adverse reactions to Zoloft and Prozac. She also knew that a new anti-depressant would take close to a month to begin to have a full effect. When she discovered that the clinical trials for rTMS, a promising technique of depolarising neurons inside the brain which is less intrusive than ECT, would not begin at a neighbouring University Medical School for two months and that she might be randomly assigned to a control group not receiving the treatment, she decided to try ECT.

Sylvia's reading, patients who had previously had the treatment and her psychiatrist supported her decision. While intrusive, ECT seemed to be more effective than psychotherapy and tricyclic antidepressants and have an overall efficacy rate of 78 per cent for individuals with her condition (Janicak *et al.* 1997: 357–87). Indeed, she reported that her psychiatrist had told her: 'In my clinical practice I have had about an 80 per cent success rate with patients like you'. Given all of these facts and her sense of urgency, Sylvia decided to begin an immediate course of ECT after talking it over with her husband.

At this point, her psychiatrist called the hospital to arrange for a series of ECT treatments and, at the request of Sylvia and her husband, called the patient's insurance company for approval of the procedure according to the rules of her insurance plan. The insurance company representative pre-certified the ECT series only as an outpatient procedure and would not put the pre-approval in writing. Sylvia's husband asked for the name of the insurance company representative, called him, waited in queue for 16 minutes 'on hold' on a telephone answering system and finally questioned him about this pre-certification procedure. He reported that the representative had responded on 19 September 1998, 'We will not pay for inpatient ECT under any conditions because those services are more expensive and not appropriate for the patient's condition. Your pre-assigned certification number does not mean that we will pay for all or part of the procedure. But, you will have a better chance of being covered, if you take the outpatient option'. Under these conditions, Sylvia and her husband were deeply worried about her health and elected to proceed with outpatient treatment. However, Sylvia's husband, unnerved by the process, began to keep a complete diary of all events related to the treatment.

Sylvia began her ECT treatment on 14 October 1998 and subsequently had two treatments a week for two-and-a-half weeks. After each treatment in the morning and a few hours of observation in the hospital, her husband took her home to rest and recover with no medical support to contact for help except during the regular 9–5 business hours, Monday to Friday. She stopped the treatment after the fifth session because she experienced intense pain in her jaws, disorienting memory loss and, finally, inability to sleep at all for three days. Many of these symptoms could have been easily handled in an inpatient setting, but the patient often experienced these symptoms at night and on week-ends when there was effectively no medical help available. After failing in this course of treatment, Sylvia became even more depressed. Her husband adjusted his work schedule to be home with her as much as possible during this recovery period. Seeking relief, her psychiatrist put her on a new anti-depressant, Remeron, which ultimately alleviated her symptoms by March 1999. After this series of events, Sylvia reported her psychiatrist saying to her: 'I hate how the practice of medicine has changed. I know what my patients need but often the insurance won't pay for the right treatment so, like my colleagues, I might have to begin to bend the rules to care for my patients'. She was referring to physicians who manipulate insurance company rules or use deception in favour of patients to be able to deliver what they deem to be appropriate care (Editorial 1999, Simon et al. 1999, Wynia et al. 2000).

Later Sylvia and her husband learned that inpatient treatment was more expensive but about 40–50 per cent more effective than the outpatient treatment that had failed. This is because side effects can be managed well in the hospital and the patient can receive three treatments per week rather than two. But, managed care organisations encourage outpatient treatment to save costs even though this procedure is less efficacious. This obvious rationing mechanism is seemingly driven by cost control and individual physician and corporation profits, not by quality of care and the likely treatment outcomes.

Another wave of unanticipated rationing mechanisms were applied to Sylvia and her husband when they attempted in 'good faith' to settle the medical bills associated with treatment for this episode. Sylvia's husband took on these problems as discussion of the complexity and size of the bills, about $11,000, added to Sylvia's depression. First, the hospital billed the patient's health insurance company but provided no itemised details. The psychiatrist and anaesthesiologists also independently billed the insurance company. All payments were denied with no explanation from the insurance company on computer-generated rejection notices. After seven telephone calls (often waiting in a queue for up to 18 minutes only to be given another number to call) and letters to physicians, the hospital billing office, three different anaesthesiologists, insurance companies and the employer that provided the benefits, Sylvia's husband reported that: (1) the telephone contact system was designed to 'cool out' the patient and make contact difficult so that the patient would just settle the bill without discussion; (2) the physicians did not want to discuss bills so referred any questions about charges or payment to their business office managers or the insurance companies; (3) physicians and the insurance company did not respond to letters; (4) entry level hospital employees in the hospital billing office and at the insurance company only read their 'rules' to the caller, making any discussion of the bill difficult; and, (5) only supervisors and upper level managers had the authority to do much more than communicate, 'you may pay your bill now or we will take action later', implying that the bill would ultimately be sent to collections, if not paid soon.

After finally reaching supervisors in the hospital billing office and insurance company, Sylvia's husband discovered that the employee's health insurance company ('Corporate Health', a pseudonym) had recently sub-contracted all mental health claims to a separate managed care firm without clearly informing employees of this action. Therefore, all mental health claims had to be sent to the second managed care firm ('Green Pastures', another pseudonym). The first round of claims was therefore sent to the wrong firm by the hospital and physicians, and in insufficient detail so they were summarily denied by Corporate Health with no explanation. After clearing up this fact, Sylvia's husband asked all the parties to bill Green Pastures. Sylvia's psychiatrist had previously established a personal relationship with a managed care supervisor at Green Pastures so she called this contact, explained the situation and asked to be paid. The supervisor immediately approved the psychiatrist's payment. The three different anaesthesiologists charged between $275 and $455 for the same procedure delivered on five separate occasions. Two of the anaesthesiologists were paid at a rate of $273 per procedure. The third anaesthesiologist and the hospital bill of $7700 were not paid in the first submission or on appeal because a Green Pastures case manager said: 'The services were not authorised and were not needed for the diagnosis'. In the meantime, the billing offices of the anaesthesiologists and the hospital continued to bill Sylvia and threatened to send her bills to a collection agency, if they were not paid in full.

In an effort to forestall such action, Sylvia's husband paid the anaesthesiologists in full and after many calls and holding patterns reached the top billing administrator at the hospital. The husband was caught in a bind because he had learned that if he paid the hospital in full, he was unlikely to be reimbursed for any of the $7700. The hospital billing administrator told Sylvia's husband: 'If you pay immediately, we will give you a 20 per cent discount. But, if you wait more than a month, your bill will be sent to collections'. In desperation and after many phone calls and considerable detective work, Sylvia's husband finally reached the Director of Managed Care for Green Pastures on his mobile phone. Sylvia's husband had asked the physicians and hospital for itemised bills of all procedures and finally received them and had his diary, which included the telephone semi-approval of the treatment. He reviewed all this with the Director and noted that Green Pastures had approved the payment to the psychiatrist and for part of the anaesthesiologists' bills. The Director quickly reviewed this history on his computerised database. Sylvia's husband reported that he spoke rapidly in summarising the case:

> We are in business to make money. Some patients try to consume more or more expensive services than they need so we have systems to control these costs. But, the doctors and hospitals are also out for themselves. They want to maximise their incomes. For example, we have an agreement with your hospital to pay them 75 per cent of the billed costs and have an understanding with them that this will cover all charges so that you will not have to pay more. They tried to get you to pay an additional 25 per cent which would be pure profit for them and against our written agreement. The anaesthesiologists are also trying to get more than the $273 per procedure that we have agreed to pay them. I will personally call the hospital and anaesthesiologists to remind them of our agreement. If you have any more problems with them, call me on my mobile phone. The psychiatrist was billed and was paid according to our agreement. If you don't watch these characters, they will rob you blind.

Within three days, the billing manager at the hospital called the husband to report that Green Pastures had paid the bill and within three weeks the billing offices of the over-charging anaesthesiologists sent Sylvia a refund for the excess.

The dynamics of this case illustrate how the person in need of mental health services experiences distress, seeks help, and makes decisions about treatment, how appropriate treatment is determined and how the reimbursement system works. It is important to note that Sylvia had adequate private insurance, a college education, management skills and a supportive husband. Even with these resources, Sylvia did not receive the care she needed and the payment process took over 14 months, involved long hours of work during business hours and considerable energy to resolve under stressful conditions. The question arises: what happens to those without these resources (Iezzoni 1999)?

Case two

The single medical event in Steve's case happened as he experienced difficulty breathing while he was working at home on his computer in March 1998.

His wife was at work so there was no one else at home. As his breathing became increasingly laboured, he grew worried and called his primary care physician who told him to go immediately to a prominent, research-oriented university hospital, (University Hospital, UH, a pseudonym) where he had been previously treated for other problems. Steve called for an ambulance and phoned his wife before he left for the hospital to tell her what had happened. Since she was not in her office, he left a voice mail message. When he arrived at the hospital, he was immediately checked in, was taken to a pulmonary medicine ward, examined by a resident and put in a private room on oxygen purportedly to improve his breathing with no monitoring to check his condition.

Most survivors with post-polio syndrome (PPS) are now between the ages of 45 and 60, and younger medical staff usually are not experienced in seeing polio or in treating patients with PPS. Individuals with PPS are likely to have a reduced muscle mass, be overweight, have scoliosis, experience respiratory disorders, use wheelchairs for mobility and have a high frequency of secondary chronic conditions such as hypertension, high cholesterol and heart disease (Bach and Gombus 1990). As a consequence of these inter-related conditions, giving oxygen therapy to PPS patients often decreases ventilation, increases blood carbon dioxide (CO_2) levels and can lead to people stopping breathing completely (Bach and Tilton 1997). Drugs with muscle-relaxing properties and anaesthesia that depresses respiration may also be life threatening for a person with PPS. Nurses, residents and attending physicians need to know that their patients have PPS, the associated risks and how to treat them, or the PPS patient will be in danger of death or increased disability. Steve was in some ways a typical case of PPS. He had compromised pulmonary function, was overweight, had scoliosis, used a wheelchair for mobility and smoked heavily.

Steve reported that the resident who initially saw him knew very little about PPS, assumed that he was a paraplegic with a respiratory problem, did not take an adequate medical history, ask him about his medical problems or how he was dealing with them. Neither did he call his primary care physician nor consult at that time with the attending physician. As a consequence, the physician embarked on a dangerous course of action.

Steve's wife reported that as soon as she spoke with her husband and realised what was going on, she immediately asked to speak to an attending physician to explain the risks of this course of action. Simultaneous with this conversation, Steve began to stop breathing. He was instantly taken to the Intensive Care Unit (ICU) where he was 'coded', meaning judged to be in danger of death. At that point, Steve's wife called his son in California and they both rushed to the hospital to take a very active role in managing Steve's care. One of his lungs had collapsed. Steve did not need oxygen but needed to be put on a ventilator, which soon happened. At this point, Steve's wife reported that the medical staff were so concerned about his being in heightened distress over being on a ventilator, not realising that he used one every night, that they heavily sedated him for six days in the ICU. This effectively removed him from any knowledge of or participation in his treatment decisions. While in the ICU, he was rarely checked and in fact the blood pressure monitor in his room did not work. During the time while he was unconscious, not fully understanding the nature of PPS or his scoliosis, the medical staff gave him an x-ray, which they could not clearly read, but still proceeded to stretch him out into a "normal" position which caused nerve damage that persists to this day.

Interviews with medical staff by Steve and his wife after the event, revealed that the staff were not knowledgeable on PPS, they did not communicate clearly among themselves nor have contact with Steve's primary care physician, and did not want the wife, son or Steve to be actively involved in the decision making or course of treatment. They were also strongly influenced by their own cultural values. Steve's wife reported that one resident said: 'Being on a ventilator is a horrible and fearful experience. Therefore we wanted to keep him heavily sedated so he would not feel distress'. The resident and attending physician had never asked Steve if he had ever been on a ventilator and felt comfortable with it. In fact, Steve used one every night and was quite comfortable with it. He said later, 'Being on a ventilator makes me feel supported; it protects you and cares for you. I certainly didn't want the tracheotomy they wanted to give me. That is much worse but we had to fight for the ventilator treatment that we knew worked and were comfortable with'. Here selection of treatment was based on staff assumptions which had not been tested on the consumer.

Interactions and further interviews with doctors, nurses and insurance company managers by Steve, his wife and the investigator revealed additional biases and pressures that influenced the rationing of care. There was an implicit assumption about quality of life on the part of the medical staff that was embedded in a nurse's comment Steve's wife reported: 'Why use high tech life support systems to prolong the lives of seriously disabled people who will have no life anyway and will be a burden on their families?' A doctor said later to the investigator about such a case: 'Why burden the family for more years?' Interestingly enough, they rarely asked the disabled person or his loved ones what they experienced and what they would have liked. Insurance companies also have a prejudice against life support systems which are expensive and likely to keep a person alive for years without what they deem to be a high quality of life. An insurance company manager said to the investigator, 'We try to make decisions on what is best for the family and on the best use of our resources for the group that we insure'.

Steve's comment about this was: 'In this situation, doctors and insurance companies only think in terms of letting you die or trashing you because you aren't worth the investment'. In Steve's case he, his wife and son presented a united front that the hospital staff did not expect, and would check to make sure that appropriate medical care was given. They knew that Steve could get back to his normal routine, if only the hospital staff would co-operate.

Then, the next controversy arose. Steve reported that the attending physician wanted to give him a permanent tracheotomy because he said to him: 'If you are intubated for more than a week, you will not be able to breathe when you come off'. Steve's wife and son knew a great deal about respiratory function and treatment because Steve had used a ventilator for years as had a number of their friends. Steve and his family insisted that he be extubated with a positive pressure nasal mask nearby in case of need. The staff finally agreed to try this and Steve breathed fine. After this experience, Steve reported that the attending physician had said: 'You had better go home now because hospitals are dangerous places to be'.

Steve was quickly discharged from the hospital without any exit strategy or training for the transition home. The hospital staff did not teach him how to use the new ventilator they prescribed, how to deal with the alarm on the machine, nor socialised him about what to expect. For most people, this raises anxiety and can even produce terror in case the alarm might go off or the person might again have difficulty breathing. Since Steve was in the hospital for almost two weeks, he lost considerable upper body strength. Upper body strength is most important for PPS individuals because they need this for transferring to and from their wheelchairs to be independent. The medical staff at the hospital said that he could get physical therapy at home. The insurance company only authorised three home visits by a physical therapist who was supposed to teach him how to do his own physical therapy.

This transition strategy did not work, leaving Steve unable to function independently, confined to bed and in danger of permanent loss of function due to premature release from the hospital, no effective discharge plan and minimal, effective physical therapy assistance offered by the insurance company. As a consequence, he contacted his primary care physician who admitted him to an excellent rehabilitation hospital (First Rate Rehab, FRR, the pseudonym used here) where he was evaluated, taught how to use his new ventilator, deal with the alarm and given eight days of physical and occupational therapy. At the point that he was able to function independently and was comfortable, FRR sent him home. From that time, Steve has been able to function independently and go back to work. Steve concluded:

This is the difference between an acute care versus rehab mentality. Although having a national reputation, UH has a fragmented system where arrogant residents saw me with breathing difficulties in a wheelchair, asked me if I could move or had any feeling in my legs, assumed that I was a paraplegic and put me on oxygen therapy without following up. This almost killed me. Polio is not the same as spinal cord injury. Since they don't know about and don't value post-polio syndrome patients, they don't go out of their way. One of my friends in her 40s who had been admitted to the hospital with pneumonia and had difficulty breathing was asked by a physician: 'Are you ready to sign a DNR when you stop breathing?' (Do Not Resuscitate Order). They didn't even tell her about her options. She died from suffocation when her respirator failed at a change of shifts in the hospital. The insurance company all but told me 'You won't get more treatment or physical therapy because you aren't worth it'. Are we outliving our welcome? Are some qualities of life not worth living in their eyes? 'A stroke, huh. Do you want a DNR?' When you are in that situation, you don't know if your wishes are being carried out. You are told indirectly or often not so subtly that they don't care much about you and that you are not a good investment. The problems are the value of your life and their perceived return on investment.

Steve's experiences with his insurance company mirror those of Sylvia's in many ways. He also spent over a year settling all accounts. He had the same problems in reaching decision makers, holding on the telephone for hours, getting clear explanations of benefits, finding out what and how much the insurance company paid, never being called back after leaving messages and having to pay doctors, hospitals and medical supply companies under threat of having his bills sent to collection.

When Steve called one of the doctors to discuss why the physician had charged more than what he had agreed with the insurance company as being 'reasonable and customary', the doctor refused to speak directly with him, but the bill was adjusted and the excess charges disappeared. He reported that when he asked doctors and hospitals for itemised bills, he received statements with charges for coded procedures; sometimes including over 20 procedures a day. When he asked for a copy of the coding manual or an explanation so that he could calculate what he was paying for, they refused to do so but significantly adjusted his charges lower. When he discovered errors in billing, it was almost always in favour of the provider or insurance company. Steve commented, 'I learned that profit was part of their organisational culture but not necessarily integrated care'. This activity took days of work over months but saved thousands of dollars. Finally, after months of work, personal payment of thousands of dollars of bills and continual battles, he unexpectedly received a refund check for $5500 from one of the hospitals. After considerable soul searching, he and his wife concluded that if they were to send the cheque to their insurance company, they would never see it. If they were to ask the hospital or insurance company for an explanation, it would take hours of work and they would lose the money, so they kept it. Steve's wife concluded from this experience:

This is a war about money and power. They do everything they can to discourage empowerment. For once, a disabled person won something against the giants in a fight. What does this encourage? Certainly not working together towards an equitable integrated or reasonably priced health care system.

Discussion and conclusion

These two cases illustrate the interaction of complex historical, structural, cultural, social and moral forces operating in the American health care system. They also highlight the cognitive frameworks of the major decision makers in American health care at the point of contact (Ross and Albrecht 2000). But most importantly, these two cases demonstrate the political economic forces at work on the micro level in the rationing of care and resources in the disability arena. The lack of knowledge and experience of many physicians with conditions like post-polio syndrome, the inability of many physicians to recognise depression in their patients, a rush through the basic facts of a case and making of unwarranted assumptions without checking them out with the patients and families, coupled with an imperative to intervene quickly with high technology solutions, constitutes a decision-making environment designed to keep the physician in control, reduce time per case, maximise profits and income and produce serious shortcomings or even mistakes in patient care. The fragmented nature of the care system and lack of integration between the component parts of complex systems for disabled people insures that consistent, quality outcomes in patient care and efficient use of resources are unlikely to happen (Williams and Bury 1989, Bury 2000b).

The reasons for this are multiple. Physician training focuses on technically measurable organic conditions, what is current and, in the context of a high-tech, post-industrial society, on acute episodes of specific diseases, is dismissive of much mental illness and does not teach critical communication skills with patients, families and insurance company representatives. In sum, doctors are taught and have incentives to deal with the patient out of context. From a political economic perspective, there are perverse incentives that discourage stakeholders from taking the time to gather a full history of their patients and from co-operating in planning and delivering care as a team.

In analysing the two cases presented above, it is imperative to recognise that no one was really in charge. Care in these instances was fragmented because there was little incentive to co-operate and collaborate and the organisational structure served to keep it that way. Steve's wife commented, 'We saw that primary care doctors were often not part of the patient's care team, not asked for information or advice nor informed of their patient's condition and progress'. As Steve remarked, 'Once you are in the hospital, your regular doctor is not your doctor and you aren't even supposed to talk to him. And it was clear that my doctors never talked to each other. When you are moved from one service to another, someone else is in charge'. In such a system, no one has complete or even good information. Each stakeholder group focuses on its own financial interests and narrowly defined area of expertise (Makover 1998). No one is responsible for the 'whole patient' or making sense of the 'big picture'. As a consequence, each time that a patient enters or exits a treatment environment, mistakes and inefficient behaviour are likely to occur, compromising the outcome of patient care and frequently driving up costs.

These problems of control and co-ordination are reinforced at every level in the political economic system. Physicians are trained as professionals to maintain control over their work and decisions, focus on their specialty, realise that they are paid by patient volume and utilisation of expensive procedures and evaluated by whether they provided care according to the 'book'. The 'book' can be guidelines for clinical services, steps in addressing specific medical conditions or running their practice according to the rules of the managed care organisation and insurance companies designed to control costs and maximise profits. Most physicians share the value of doing what is best for the patient but this can be interpreted in various ways by the group practice, hospital, insurance company, medical school administration, patients and their families. As we have seen, many physicians now feel compelled to make alternative diagnoses, bend the rules and generally manipulate the system to produce what they in conscience and by training know to be right for the patient.

The irony is that the potential quality and efficiency of care in this system is high, causing many non-disabled people to say: 'This is the best health care system in the world'. Disabled people remark that these individuals have never had a disability and had to deal with the reality of the system. Most of the necessary component pieces are in place but no one is managing the whole system. In fact, the participating stakeholders have obvious conflicts of interest in terms of money and power that subvert the general system goals.

The mechanisms for rationing care are myriad and complex but in most cases are designed to maximise the interests of a single stakeholder or coalition of institutional stakeholders. The stakeholders with most power tend to win. Physicians have traditionally had the power of knowledge and a guild. This is moderated today by the countervailing power of managers in the corporations where doctors now tend to work, and in those insurance companies and managed care corporations that control their incomes and work conditions; physician group practices, for-profit hospital chains, community hospital corporations, university health science centres and government agencies (Bodenheimer and Casalino 1999, Banja and DeJong 2000). The mechanisms for rationing care can be explicit as in the case of the Oregon Health Plan (Bodenheimer 1997), or implicit as Mechanic (1995) advocates. Neither system seems to have the best interests of disabled people at heart. Rationing of care takes place on two levels: (1) the amount and type of care received including access, knowledge of what is possible and available, offering participation to the disabled person in the decision making, the subjective calculation of value of life, decisions to make no further effort to prolong life or preserve levels of functional independence, limitations to high technology care and assistive devices, modification of the home environment to permit independent living and integrated care managers who can help navigate the transitions and problems; and (2) the powerful control of billing, reimbursement rules, criteria for making reimbursement decisions, access to billing information and detailed accounting, norms of what are customary and reasonable charges. There are also the inordinate layers of bureaucracy that must be navigated to receive reimbursement, the length of time from billing to reimbursement (often requiring the patient to be the 'bank' for the system), the hidden contracts between providers and insurers and the propensity for providers to pressure patients to pay more out of pocket than agreed upon to increase the profits of doctors and hospitals.

As is clear in the two cases above, the only effective care managers for the patients' best interests were the patients themselves and their families. There is limited accountability (Millenson 1999). The patient has little power, expertise, legal recourse or resources to unravel the behind-the-scenes agreements that constitute a care system designed to use the patient for profit. The major stakeholders in this micro-political economic system have wellbeing as a goal, but most often their own wellbeing takes precedence over that of patients and their families. The present versions of rationed care health care systems found in developed countries disproportionately vest power in the hands of medical professionals, pharmaceutical and medical supply companies, insurance corporations, hospitals and health centres and the government. Established laws and practice patterns reinforce this power imbalance. As a consequence, the structure, practice and outcomes of health care systems are determined by the powerful institutional stakeholders; not by the consumer, citizen or patient (Hughes *et al.* 1997). The practice of medicine, therefore, reflects and reinforces established stratification systems where the most desirable goods and services are reserved for those who have money and connections. That is why health care remains a major fault line in Western democratic societies for it calls into question how the values of equality and concern for citizens are enacted in the political economic system.

References

Albrecht, G.L. (1992) *The Disability Business: Rehabilitation in America.* Thousand Oaks, CA: Sage.

Albrecht, G.L. and Bury, M. (2001) The political economy of the disability marketplace. In Albrecht, G.L., Seelman, K. and Bury, M. (eds) *Handbook of Disability Studies.* Thousand Oaks, CA: Sage.

Albrecht, G.L. and Devlieger, P.J. (1999) The disability paradox: high quality of life against all odds, *Social Science and Medicine*, 48, 977–88.

Albrecht, G.L. and Verbrugge, L.M. (2000) The global emergence of disability. In Albrecht, G.L., Fitzpatrick, R. and Scrimshaw, S.C. (eds) *Handbook of Social Studies in Health and Medicine.* London: Sage.

Alt, J.E. and Alesina, A. (1996) Political economy: an overview. In Goodin, R.E. and Klingemann, H.D. (eds) *A New Handbook of Political Science*. New York: Oxford University Press.

Altman, B. (2001) Disability definitions, models, classification schemes, and applications. In Albrecht, G.L., Seelman, K.S. and Bury, M. (eds) *Handbook of Disability Studies*. Thousand Oaks, CA: Sage.

Bach, J. and Gombus, G. (1990) Quality of life perceptions of ventilator-assisted individuals, *IVUN News*, 4, 1–2.

Bach, J.R. and Tilton, M. (1997) Pulmonary dysfunction and its management in post-polio patients, *NeuroRehabilitation*, 8, 139–53.

Banja, J.D. and DeJong, G. (2000) The rehabilitation marketplace: economics, values, and proposals for reform, *Archives of Physical Medicine and Rehabilitation*, 81, 233–40.

Beedle, D., Krasuski, J. and Janicak, P.G. (1998) Advances in somatic therapies: electroconvulsive therapy, repetitive transcranial magnetic stimulation, and bright light therapy. In Janicak, P.G. (ed) *Update: Principles and Practice of Psychopharmacotherapy 2nd Edition*. Baltimore: Williams and Wilkins.

Bodenheimer, T. (1997) The Oregon health plan – lessons for the nation, *The New England Journal of Medicine*, 337, 720–3.

Bodenheimer, T. and Casalino, L. (1999) Executives with white coats – the work and world view of managed-care medical directors, *The New England Journal of Medicine*, 341, 2029–32.

Brudevold, C., McGhee, S.M. and Ho, L.M. (2000) Contract medicine arrangements in Hong Kong: an example of risk-bearing provider networks in an unregulated environment, *Social Science and Medicine*, 51, 1221-9.

Bury, M. (2000a) A comment on the ICIDH2, *Disability and Society*, 15, 1073–7.

Bury, M.R. (2000b) Health ageing and the lifecourse. In Williams, S.J., Gabe, J. and Calnan, M. (eds) *Health, Medicine and Society: Key Theories, Future Agendas*. London: Routledge.

Castel, R. (1995) *Les métaphorphoses de la question sociale*. Paris: Fayard.

Centers for Disease Control (2000) *Healthy People 2010*. Atlanta, GA: Centers for Disease Control.

Charmaz, K. (1991) *Good Days, Bad Days: The Self in Chronic Illness and Time*. New Brunswick, NJ: Rutgers University Press.

Charmaz, K. (2000) Experiencing chronic illness. In Albrecht, G.L., Fitzpatrick, R. and Scrimshaw, S.C. (eds) *Handbook of Social Studies in Health and Medicine*. London: Sage.

Commission Europeene (2000) Reconstituter les corps blessés, *Cordis Focus*, 149, 1–2.

Dudley, R.A., Miller, R.H., Korenbrot, T.Y. and Luft, H.S. (1998) The impact of financial incentives on quality of health care. *Milbank Quarterly*, 76, 649–86.

Druss, B.G., Schlesinger, M., Thomas, T. and Allen, H. (2000) Chronic illness and plan satisfaction under managed care, *Health Affairs*, 19, 203–9.

Editorial (1999) Care of patients and subterfuge, in equal parts, *Lancet*, 354, 1743.

Eist, H.I. (1998) Treatment for major depression in managed care and fee-for-service systems, *The American Journal of Psychiatry*, 155, 859–60.

Evans, R.G. (1984) *Strained Mercy: the Economics of Canadian Health Care*. Toronto: Butterworths.

Fink, M. (1999) *Electroshock: Restoring the Mind*. New York: Oxford University Press.

Garvey, J.V. (1993) Health-care rationing and the Americans with Disabilities Act of 1990 – what protection should the disabled be afforded? *Notre Dame Law Review*, 68, 581–617.

Griffiths, L. and Hughes, D. (1998) Purchasing in the British NHS: does contracting mean explicit rationing? *Health*, 2, 349–71.

Handwerker, W.P. and Borgatti, S.P. (1998) Reasoning with numbers. In Bernard, H.R. (ed) *Handbook of Methods in Cultural Anthropology*. Walnut Creek, CA: Altamira Press.

Harris, G.E., Ripperger, M.J. and Horn, H.G. (2000) Managed care at a crossroads, *Health Affairs*, 19, 163.

Harrison, S. and Moran, M. (2000) Resources and rationing: managing supply and demand in health care. In Albrecht, G.L., Fitzpatrick, R. and Scrimshaw, S.C. (eds) *Handbook of Social Studies in Health and Medicine*. London: Sage.

Hedlund, M. (2000) Disability as a phenomenon: a discourse of social and bio-medical understanding, *Disability and Society*, 15, 765–80.

Hornbrook, M. and Goodman, M. (1996) Chronic disease, functional health states, and demographics: a multi-dimensional approach to risk adjustment, *Health Services Research*, 31, 283–307.

Hughes, D., Griffiths, L. and McHale, J.V. (1997) Do quasi-markets evolve? Institutional analysis and the NHS, *Cambridge Journal of Economics*, 21, 259–76.

Iezoni, L. (1999) Boundaries. What happens to the disabled poor when insurers draw a line between what's 'medically necessary' and devices that can improve quality of life? *Health Affairs*, 18, 171–6.

Janicak, P., Davis, J.M., Preskorn, S.H. and Ayd, Jr., F.J. (1997) *Principles and Practice of Psychopharmacotherapy* 2nd Edition. Baltimore, MD: Williams and Williams.

Jensen, G.A., Morrisey, M.A., Gaffney, S. and Liston, D.K. (1997) The new dominance of managed care: insurance trends in the 1990s, *Health Affairs*, 16, 126–36.

Light, D.W. (1992) The practice and ethics of risk-rated health insurance, *Journal of the American Medical Association*, 267, 2503–8.

Light, D.W. (1995) *Health Care Reform: Lessons from the British Experience*. Washington, D.C.: Physician Payment Review Commission.

Light, D.W. (2000) The sociological character of health-care markets. In Albrecht, G.L., Fitzpatrick, R. and Scrimshaw, S.C. (eds) *Handbook of Social Studies in Health and Medicine*. London: Sage.

Llewellyn, A. and Hogan, K. (2000) The use and abuse of models of disability, *Disability and Society*, 15, 157–65.

Luft, H. and Miller, R. (1988) Patient selection in a competitive health care system, *Health Affairs*, 97–119.

Makover, M.E. (1998) *Mismanaged Care: How Corporate Medicine Jeopardizes Your Health*. Amhert, N.Y.: Prometheus Books.

Mechanic, D. (1995) Dilemmas in rationing health care services: the case for implicit rationing, *British Medical Journal*, 310, 1655–61.

Mehlman, M.J., Durshslag, M.R. and Neuhauser, D. (1997) When do health care decisions discriminate against persons with disabilities? *Journal of Health Politics, Policy and Law*, 22, 1385–411.

Millenson, M.L. (1999) *Demanding Medical Excellence: Doctors and Accountability In the Information Age*. Chicago: University of Chicago Press.

Miller, W.L. and Crabtree, B.F. (2000) Clinical research. In Denzin, N.K. and Lincoln, Y.S. (eds) *Handbook of Qualitative Research*, 2nd Edition. Thousand Oaks, CA: Sage.

Murray, C.J. and Lopez, A.M. (eds) (1996) *The Global Burden of Disease*. Boston, MA: Harvard University Press.

Pfeiffer, D. (2000) The devils are in the details: the ICIDH2 and the disability movement, *Disability and Society*, 15, 1079–82.

Rier, D.A. (2000) The missing voice of the critically ill: a medical sociologist's first-person account, *Sociology of Health and Illness*, 22, 68–93.

Ross, J. and Albrecht, G.L. (2000) Understanding and managing health care intervention for the terminally ill, *Research in the Sociology of Health Care*, 17, 3–29.

Scheier, L. (2000) Access denied: people with pre-existing medical conditions languish in health insurance limbo, *Chicago Tribune*, 5 May, 1, 5.

Seymour, W. (1998) *Remaking the Body: Rehabilitation and Change*. London: Routledge.

Simon, S.R., Pan, R.J., Sullivan, A.M., Clark-Chiarelli, N., Connelly, M.T., Peters, A.S., Singer, J.D., Inui, T.S. and Block, S.D. (1999) Views of managed care: a survey of students, residents, faculty, and deans of medical schools in the United States, *The New England Journal of Medicine*, 340, 928–36.

Stake, R.E. (2000) Case studies. In Denzin, N.K. and Lincoln, Y.S. (eds) *Handbook of Qualitative Research*, 2nd Edition. Thousand Oaks, CA: Sage.

Stocker, K., Waitzkin, H. and Iriat, C. (1999) The exportation of managed care to Latin America, *The New England Journal of Medicine*, 340, 1131–36.

Stone, D.A. (1988) *The Disabled State*. Philadelphia: Temple University Press.

Stone, D.A. (1993) The struggle for the soul of health insurance, *Journal of Health Politics, Policy and Law*, 18, 287–317.

Strauss, A. (1993) *Continual Permutations of Action*. New York: Aldine De Gruyter.

Thorne, S.E. (1993) *Negotiating Health Care: The Social Context of Chronic Illness*. Newbury Park, CA: Sage.

Williams, G.H. (2001) Theorizing disability. In Albrecht, G.L., Seelman, K.S. and Bury, M. (eds) *Handbook of Disability Studies*. Thousand Oaks, CA: Sage.

Williams, S.J. and Bury, M.R. (1989) Impairment, disability and handicap in chronic respiratory illness, *Social Science and Medicine*, 29, 609–16.

Wynia, M.K., Cummins, D.S., VanGeest, J.B. and Wilson, I.B. (2000) Physician manipulation of reimbursement rules for patients, *Journal of the American Medical Association*, 283, 1858–65.

7

Categorising to exclude: the discursive construction of cases in community mental health teams

Lesley Griffiths

Introduction

This chapter examines data from meetings in which social workers and nurses in British community mental health teams (CMHTs) process referrals from consultant psychiatrists and GPs, and decide whether or not patients should be 'allocated' to team members. The starting point is the observation that CMHTs face a recurrent problem of prioritising some patient referrals for attention, while not accepting others onto staff caseloads. In contrast to the situation in the 1960s, when many commentators complained of the excessive use of psychiatric diagnoses and compulsory institutionalisation, community-based mental health services in the 1990s had become a scarce resource not available to all patients. In recent years official policy has increasingly sought to direct CMHTs to target the 'seriously mentally ill', while leaving primary care to provide for patients with less serious conditions (DoH 1994, Audit Commission 1994). This posed difficulties in the new internal market environment, in which funding streams were partially dependent on referrals from primary care doctors, which often involved non-psychotic conditions. Thus Tredget and Bowler (2000: 48) comment that many CMHTs find themselves 'dancing to two distinct drums: the policy-driven rhythm of the health authority, focusing on people with serious mental illness, and the previously market-driven rhythm of the PHCT (primary health care team), prioritising people with less severe problems' (see also: Shears and Coleman, 1999). Against a background of heavy workloads, a move towards targeting the seriously mentally ill, inevitably translates into less care for other groups. As Shepherd (1995: 15) observes, this means de facto rationing, whether through outright denial of access to specialist services, or limitation or delay of such access.

The analysis focuses on the discursive construction of cases, and the way in which some patients are marked out by rank-and-file team members as inappropriate referrals in a process of implicit categorisation that generally avoids open reference to alternative diagnostic labels. My argument is that rationing in this context is affected by global issues of resources and demand, but also by struggles between the different professionals within the CMHT who attempt to draw the boundaries of patient eligibility in ways that suit their interests. Rationing becomes entwined with concerns about workload pressures and funding, as well as ongoing negotiations about the nature of CMHTs, teamwork and occupational identities. Although team members generally cast their discussions in terms of appropriateness rather than rationing, they openly link the former to the need for 'gatekeeping' and make frequent references to limited resources. The need to exclude some patients to limit workload forms a taken-for-granted backdrop to discourse in team meetings, which is often in tension with the more inclusive approach favoured by the psychiatrist-manager. There is a process of categorisation in which patients are located as falling inside or outside the target group for community mental health services, which effectively defines the boundaries of mental illness. While eligibility for CMHT services generally depends on categorising patients in terms of formal psychiatric diagnoses or their organisational variants (*explicit labelling*), non-eligibility is typically signalled in a more elliptical way by constructing a picture of the case in terms other than 'serious mental illness' (*implicit categorisation*). I shall argue that this indirect approach to categorisation allows team members to oppose the psychiatrist's or GP's referral without requiring that any individual mounts an explicit challenge: an alternative definition of the case emerges a step at a time in the context of a group discussion.

A more general concern of the chapter is to illustrate the complexities that surround categorisation and selection processes in human service organisations. One unfortunate legacy of sociological labelling theory was that it focused attention on the social significance of naming, and diverted attention away from the face-to-face interactions from which 'labels' emerged. Although there is a growing literature on the micro-level practices of categorisation in institutional settings (Hak 1998, Heritage and Lindstrom 1998, Antaki 2001), too many medical sociologists still operate with impoverished conceptions of categorisation, in which the emphasis remains on explicit labelling rather than processes of implicit categorisation of the kind described here. This chapter will provide a further illustration of categorisation in action, which will give due weight to its subtlety and its close connection with contextual influences. After describing the research methods, I shall discuss CMHT members' preoccupation with resources and the need for better gatekeeping of referrals, and then examine the nature of patient categorisation and selection. I describe how rank-and-file staff's attempts to screen out a proportion of patients is cast in the language of 'inappropriateness', how staff challenge psychiatrists' expert diagnoses with alternative formulations that 'normalise' patients' conditions, and how far psychiatrists are able to enforce a more inclusive referral policy in the face of team resistance.

The study and the setting

This chapter discusses previously unpublished aspects of a study of two Welsh community mental health teams carried out in the mid-1990s (Griffiths 1996, 1997, 1998). These newly-established teams were affected by two major policy developments that shaped the environment in which they had to function. CMHTs were a key element in the community care policies set out in the 1991 All Wales Strategy for Mental Health, which were intended to take mental health services outside the hospitals and change relationships between the NHS and social services. But they came into being against the background of the 1991 NHS internal market reforms, which transformed patterns of funding, and required that services such as CMHTs generated sufficient contractual income to justify their existence. Each CMHT was led by a psychiatrist, with combined clinical and management responsibilities, and comprised community psychiatric nurses (CPNs)[1] and social workers. One team had rooms both at a local psychiatric hospital and the social services department area offices; the second had accommodation in a local health centre and at the area offices.

The work of the CMHTs includes community-based treatment and support of patients and their families, assessment of new cases and the management of psychiatric emergencies. The focus of the research, however, was on collegial interaction between members of the newly-constituted teams, and particularly on weekly team meetings in which cases were discussed. In one CMHT (Team A) these meetings ostensibly focused on the task of the 'allocation' of new patients to the caseloads of individual team members; in the other (Team B) they were described as 'review' meetings, in which team members were expected to discuss their management of patients. Actually, the distinction was less clear-cut than these designations might suggest, since allocation meetings might include the review of some difficult cases, and review meetings might touch on new cases allocated to team members at that meeting. Team A meetings were not attended by the psychiatrist, and referrals were introduced by the nurse manager or social worker team leader, who alternated as chairperson. The Team B psychiatrist chaired the weekly meetings and played an active role in discussions about patients.

The research was conceived as an organisational ethnography, which however would pay special attention to language use, and combine participant observation with analysis of the organisation of talk in the weekly team meetings. Following a period of initial non-participant observation, twelve successive (multi-case) meetings for each team were tape-recorded and transcribed, and these form the main corpus of data for analysis. Subsequently, background interviews with all team members were completed. Permission for the study was obtained from senior health and social services staff, and then from individual team members. All were advised of the general aims of the study, of the intention to make observations and tape recordings of meetings, and of their right not to participate, but no person declined to take part. While it may have had subtle effects, the use of the tape recorder did not appear to result in major changes of behaviour: the business of categorisation proceeded and there were few indications of any attempt to self-censure comments about service users.

Transcripts of meetings were analysed inductively, attending to both their sequential organisation and their content. The transcripts were coded thematically with the aim of developing some general propositions about issues such as the division of labour, the significance of hierarchy and differential expertise, the role of humour, the versions of teamwork espoused, and the approach to categorising service users, and illustrative data extracts were identified. The longer extracts were also analysed in terms of their sequential organisation, and what this revealed about the social organisation of team meetings. Where cases or team issues were discussed over more than one meeting, the relevant sections of transcripts were read in chronological order, and attempts were made to contextualise particular data extracts in terms of these ongoing discussions. All proper names in transcripts are pseudonyms.

Workload pressures, gatekeeping and buffering

I argued in an earlier paper that CMHTs are an arena for occupational conflict about the nature of mental health work and the definition of the client group (Griffiths, 1997). My data contain many examples of definitional struggles between psychiatrists, operating with relatively inclusive nosologies of psychopathology, and social workers, who see many presenting problems as 'a normal reaction to life events'[2]. This line of division was accentuated by different perspectives on the recent NHS reforms and their resource implications. Where psychiatrist/managers were concerned to demonstrate a workload for CMHTs in a competitive, market-oriented NHS, rank-and-file team members were more preoccupied with heavy caseloads, which affected them more than the referring doctors.

Average caseloads were slightly higher in Team B than in Team A, comprising around 30–50 service users per team member at any one time. The work associated with a given caseload depended in part on the type of support provided to patients. Both teams divided community mental health work into a number of activities involving more or less contact with service users. At the less demanding end of the spectrum were patients receiving regular injections at clinics, but no home visits or other support. At an intermediate level, both CMHTs ran weekly anxiety management classes (which discussed general approaches to stress management) and relaxation classes (which taught specific relaxation techniques). Both teams also organised a weekly social club, which aimed to improve patients' social skills. Many patients attending classes or the clubs received no other support but were included in caseloads. The major burden came from the group of clients who were judged to need regular home visits, counselling and other support. Some of these also attended classes and the club.

The policy in both teams was that, as far as possible, all team members were generalists, so that individual team members had mixed caseloads including patients with a range of conditions. The major exception was that patients requiring drug injections were allocated to CPNs rather than social workers. As far as could be determined, however, team members had accepted the generalist role and I found no evidence that patients of particular types were being allocated to 'unofficial' specialists.

Three main strategies were available to team members to attenuate work pressures. Firstly, some limited remission might be gained by channelling patients towards the less intensive treatment options (for example, anxiety management classes rather than home visits) or services provided by other agencies. Secondly, team members could delay the psychiatrist's referral of the patient to the CMHT, usually by requesting more information. Thirdly, the team might influence the psychiatrist or GP to reconsider the referral decision. The first two strategies represent ways of 'buffering' the team from work pressures. The third can be seen as a variety of gatekeeping. Gatekeeping is a members' concept that figured explicitly in many team meetings. Staff in both CMHTs perceived their service as a finite resource that risked being swamped by the growing demand for care.

Gatekeeping in Team B was an activity largely controlled by the psychiatrist, via his own referrals and liaison with GPs, but open to review within the team meeting and subject to some team influence. Admission decisions were more inclusionary than some team members would have liked, but were taken or confirmed after team discussions in which the impact on workload could be considered. By contrast, Team A members could influence GP referrals but lacked a direct input into the (absent) psychiatrist's gatekeeping, a role that they perceived he was not carrying out effectively. Overall, then, staff in both teams saw gatekeeping as mainly the responsibility of the psychiatrists and GPs, but themselves became involved at the margins of the process, through dialogue with the psychiatrist (Team B) or communication via the team leader with psychiatrist and GPs (Team A).

The two CMHTs approached the issue of the target user population and the management of work pressures in contrasting ways. The Team A psychiatrist attempted to construct a CMHT caseload that was relatively inclusive via the referral of significant numbers of patients with moderate depression or anxiety states. However, communication with the team was limited, and referrals were often blocked or delayed by team members. Team members were also freer to use less intensive treatment options without psychiatrist interference. The Team B psychiatrist tried to negotiate referrals on a case by case basis through his active involvement in CMHT meetings. While the team resisted some requests, the psychiatrist was generally able to get the team to accept a wider range of cases than was seen as legitimate in Team A.

Categorisation and selection

Patient selection and rationing are closely bound up with the interactional processes in which categorisations of patients are negotiated, the focus of this chapter. Categorisation and selection are analytically separate processes, so that categorisation may precede selection (and rationing) and raises issues about the boundaries of client populations that selection does not (Byrd 1981:4). In practice, however, the two activities are closely implicated. Categorisation is done not for its own sake but in order to act (Edwards, 1991), and is pragmatically linked to the 'problem relevances' and action possibilities in the particular setting (Byrd 1981: 79, Emerson 1983: 436), including limited resources and the differential resource implications of different actions.

There is now a large social science literature documenting how workers in human service agencies develop and apply typifications of the clientele to organise their work (Scheff 1965, Bloor 1976, Hughes 1976, 1980, Jeffery 1979, Kelly and May 1982, Murcott 1981, Brown 1989, Griffiths and Hughes 1993, Ashforth and Humphrey 1995). Research has shown that agency staff identify and order clients in terms of typified knowledge which defines the essential characteristics of the case and the options for action. Generally the emphasis has been on the interactional application and elaboration of typifications, so that the wider accounts of the categorisation process offered by these writers stress the importance of context and organisational environment.

CMHT members, like other human service workers, have ideas about the types of clients who present their social identities and circumstances, the underlying conditions or behaviours that lie behind the presentation, and the presence or absence of motives for observed behaviours. As Byrd (1981: 43) suggests, mental health professionals may be viewed as 'motives experts', whose task is to 'formulate the intelligibility of action when others have failed'. Case presentations tap into a rich descriptive repertoire which draws inter alia on the categories of expert psychiatric diagnosis, the more morally loaded slang of backstage medical talk, the social-psychological terms of social work discourse, and labels linked to practical perceptions of workload ('he'd be a long-term patient').

As mentioned earlier, two categories that have special significance, largely because of their recurrent use in official documents on the role of CMHTs, are the 'seriously mentally ill' and 'the worried well'. The first defines the target population for CMHTs, the second points at a group of patients who have lower priority and who do not generally require the services of the CMHT. However, these categories require situational interpretation in the light of the specifics of real cases. The following extract, comes from a Team A meeting in which participants have complained about the in-appropriateness of the referrals and the need for better 'gatekeeping'. In talking about the inappropriateness of one case, the social work team reiterates Welsh Office guidance which states that CMHTs should prioritise the serious mental illness. This is followed by an exchange that illustrates the less than straightforward nature of that category.

Extract 1

SW: I'm talking about the Welsh Office bit on it, it says about concentrating on the seriously mentally ill. But then in the next sentence it says about neuroses and milder disorders and things that the primary health care team should do. But it leaves it up in the air, you know.

SWTL: What do you mean?

SW: You sort of come away from it thinking, well I'm not quite sure really if...

SWTL: Well it's all open to interpretation, isn't it, because as far as I'm concerned, and Rory [the psychiatrist] has mentioned it a number of times, he's said, you can have people with neurotic conditions who could come under the heading of seriously mentally ill.

[Chorus of agreement from team]

SWTL: It's down to a matter of opinion on occasions.

Such problems of 'interpretation' are apparent in many other case discussions tape-recorded for the research.

The selection decisions we are considering typically occur in routinised interactions which follow a similar pattern. Medical case presentations tend to be structured as reports, constructed within a particular occupational register and conforming with certain professional norms (Anspach 1988, Poirer and Brauner 1988, Hughes and Griffiths 1996). While the nature of case presentations will vary greatly according to specialty and context, they usually comprise an account of the patient 'history' and associated events, which allows listening colleagues to make inferences about the type of case they are dealing with. They often conclude with a categorisation that is presented as emerging from the information given and/or subsequent collegial discussion. Team A allocation discussions usually start with a case presentation that has some of these features, but with the important differ-ence that it is made by a nursing or social work team leader, drawing on a referral letter (and sometimes additional written notes) supplied by the absent psychiatrist. Thus the orthodox case presentation is replaced by one made by a surrogate (one of the two team leaders), who moves between the two voices of referrer and commentator, and sometimes appears less than

fully committed to the report he is putting forward. Often, the categorisation suggested in the referral letter is probed and challenged by the listening
team members. An example from a Team A meeting follows.

Extract 2

SWTL: This patient presented with alcohol abuse and being depressed.
His appetite was fair, but he was drinking in order to sleep. He'd stopped
taking his prescribed medication and had suicidal thoughts on admission.
He'd been in [the psychiatric hospital] in the past with an inadequate
personality and depression. [starts to read from notes] Has gradually
improved and now wants to take his own discharge. He complained that
nothing had been explained to him. However, he was reluctant to accept
help. [inaudible sentence omitted] Admitted to ward A informally
following a period of disturbed behaviour. Non-compliance with
medication, drinking heavily and generally self-neglectful, referred by
neighbours who had become frightened of him, stayed for two weeks in
the hospital, discharged against medical advice. Now for follow-up
support. Early relapse anticipated, suitable for Hilltop House or a group
home. I don't know if he has stabilised, and if he is compliant with his
medication, he might be suitable for that. But this suggestion is made by
Rory [the psychiatrist], I rather suspect, and I wonder what has been
tested out on the ward with him. Ieuan, do you know?

NM: I don't know because all the time I didn't have much involvement
with him. I know that when he was on the ward he had been referred
to the rehab unit initially because there was a gap of like two or three
weeks before placement was arranged up there. I know that Rory felt that
obviously he wasn't coping in his own home, and felt that there might be a
suitable place for him to go to, go to rehab with a view to alternative
accommodation where he could be monitored. Apparently he is supposed
to be in a hell of a state.

[Three turns on details of discharge from hospital omitted. Discussion
moves on to patient's house]

NM: From there [*i.e.* the time of discharge] it was in a hell of a state.

SW1: I suspect he'll have a wad of unpaid bills. Yes, he's put in a few
windows. I don't know about Hilltop House or a group home, but I feel
that at an initial level he would be better off in a council flat. But
I wouldn't see him in Hilltop House or a group home.

SWTL: Is that because he is too good, if I can put it that way? Do you
think he is too independent?

SW1: I think on one level he could probably be very capable, couldn't he?

CPN1: Yeah I think Derek is right actually.

SWTL: Is he?

CPN1: Yeah.

SWTL: When he becomes disturbed is that due to drinking or is [he mildly sch]izophrenic =

CPN1:   [I think so]

SWTL: = or is he

SW1: There's a divorce as well isn't there?

CPN1: Yeah.

SW1: He probably needs an army of home helps to go in there because//

SWTL: Well he's had two weeks in hospital and then discharged against medical advice. It's debatable isn't it?

NM: Difficult to judge with the//

SWTL: The insinuation is that we can only help this bloke if he's prepared to accept// help

SW1: We can only offer it =

SWTL: = If he turns around and says well perhaps home help, you know in that direction.

There is some further discussion of the divorce, the blow suffered by the patient in losing his wife, and his unrealistic hope that she will come back to him, even though she has re-married. The case discussion ends with a social worker (SW1) agreeing to 'have a look' at this patient, who may then 'see some direction in which he wants to go', perhaps to return to his home country of Iran. However, no steps are taken to explore the options the psychiatrist has suggested (Hilltop House or a group home) or to arrange specific help.

The initial case presentation locates this patient as someone previously diagnosed with 'depression' and 'inadequate personality', and with recent symptoms that include depression, non-compliance with medication, 'suicidal thoughts', heavy drinking and self-neglect. He has also discharged himself 'against medical advice'. The psychiatrist has referred the patient to the CMHT for 'follow-up support', and by implication is suggesting that this diagnosis and these symptoms place the patient within the target group for the services the team offers.

One thing to notice in this extract is that team members do not challenge the psychiatric diagnosis by offering alternative diagnostic labels. Hester (1992) has suggested that references to deviance can take a number of forms. Most obviously they involve use of (a) culturally available member-ship categories, such as 'mad', or (b) type categorisations, such as 'mad type'. But reference to a deviant category can also be made less directly,

(c) by mentioning attributes culturally associated with the category, (d) by describing behaviours culturally associated with the category, (e) making comparisons with the norm, or (f) invoking more general categories such as 'trouble' or 'problem'. I want to argue that team members in the extract above are attempting an alternative framing of the reported behaviour and events, using these latter forms of referencing – mainly (c) and (d). Although Hester is writing specifically about 'deviance', I take his analysis to be applicable to most forms of categorisation in people processing organisations, and in Extract 2 it is normalisation rather than deviance that is at issue – the patient is being constructed as *not* seriously mentally ill.

We can analyse these descriptive terms as the elements which comprise membership categorisation devices. Membership categorisation is a feature of conversation originally described by Sacks (1972a, 1972b) and developed by later writers (Watson 1976, Drew 1978, Jayyusi 1984, Edwards 1991). Sacks' work on this topic is summarised by Boden:

> ... a membership categorisation device [is a] way of typifying and grouping people, objects or activities... Out of apparent chaos comes a convenient and local grouping that has a for-the-moment, just-here-and-now organization. The collection or collectivity is practical in that it solves some ongoing yet immediately relevant activity. It is a member's term in that it provides, through its construction, an inclusionary as well as exclusionary distinction which solves some local problem and, simultaneously, connects to a larger unit or set of events or people. As a categorization device, it groups the objects of the world for some relevant action or set of actions (1994: 130).

The diagnostic labels and reported symptoms (behaviours) contained in the initial case report can be read as mutually-supporting descriptive terms that make reference to the membership categorisation device of serious mental illness. In the subsequent discussion, however, team members attempt to re-order some of these elements, and introduce new elements, to point to an alternative membership categorisation device that should be considered – life problems, which fall short of serious mental illness. Early in extract 2, the social work team leader creates a space to question the case presentation he has just made, by adding the observation that it is not clear whether the recommended follow-up arrangements have been discussed with the patient. This point is emphasised by repetition: the team leader says that the recommendation has probably come from the psychiatrist, and may not have been 'tested out' with the patient in the ward. The next speaker, the nurse manager, offers no judgement on this, but maintains a sceptical stance. His comment that the patient is *'supposed to be* in a hell of a state', constructs the information coming from the psychiatrist, not as a factual report, but as an account requiring confirmatory evidence. When the discussion moves to the issue of the state of the patient's home, SW1 makes a series of references that can be heard as being more about domestic coping than about psychopathology. He mentions unpaid bills, including some for the repair of broken windows ('he's put in a few windows'), and offers the view that the patient 'would be better off in a council flat'. It is not clear whether the flat is better than the patient's present house because it is a cheaper, more manageable dwelling, or better than the group home because it will allow continuing independence. However, the social worker adds that he 'wouldn't see' the patient in the group home. This leads the team leader to ask a clarifying question about whether a group home is unsuitable because the patient is 'too good', which elicits the response that the patient 'could be very capable'. At this juncture the team leader raises the issue that the social worker may have been working towards: whether the disturbed behaviour is due to mental illness ('is he mildly schizophrenic') or to 'drinking' or something else. The placement of CPN1's answer ('I think so') suggests that she thinks drinking is the cause. SW1's statement that there is a divorce 'as well' supports the interpretation that the current problems may be due to life events rather than serious mental illness. Next, the team leader introduces the additional consideration of whether the team can help the patient if he is 'not prepared to accept' help. This has the effect of supporting the re-definition of the patient's needs as practical support rather than clinical intervention: the team leader suggests that the team can only assist 'if he turns around and says perhaps home help, you know, in that direction'.

None of the individual elements of these accounts (unpaid bills, need for a 'home help', divorce) point unequivocally towards an alternative categorisation to serious mental illness, but taken together they begin to sketch out a picture easily recognisable within the lexicon of client types known to team members. Hester (1992) argues that the recognition of deviance in referral talk routinely depends on hearing reports of the activities, attributes and problems of clients as references to their category membership. Participants are able to recognise that, even in the absence of explicit reference to a particular deviant category, repeated references to behaviours, attributes or problems conventionally associated with that deviant category, lead to the inference that it is relevant. By co-selecting terms that can be seen to 'go together', CMHT members can begin to orient the case discussion towards an alternative categorisation not pre-figured in the referral letter – a person experiencing life problems but not seriously mentally ill. It is through this 'referencing work', skilfully woven into reports and stories about service users, that definitions are contested and the boundaries between appropriate and inappropriate referrals are negotiated. A case defined as inappropriate does not require the services of the CMHT, and in this way patients with less serious psychological problems previously seen as falling within the remit of mental health services are excluded, much as Shepherd (1995) predicts.

'Does anybody know this one?'

One feature of Extract 2, not so far discussed, is that it contains segments of occupational narrative (stories of encounters with patients and other agencies), which take their authority from personal knowledge and experience rather than from expert, discipline-based knowledge. Discussions of new referrals in both teams often reach a point when the chair will invite staff accounts of past contact with patients, using some variant of 'Does anybody know this one?' Typically, such narratives are not disguised as anything other than first-person accounts[3], and communicate a version of events in which elements of formal theory may be interspersed with common-sense understandings, and facts not clearly distinguished from moral evaluations. Nevertheless, they have credibility within the team because they are based on direct contact with service users in real-life situations. Thus they may be effective as a counterpoint to observations made in the psychiatrist's referral notes, which are seen to be dependent on inferences drawn in the ward or outpatient setting and remote from 'real life'. In this way the rhetorical force of expert professional knowledge is countered by a more informal occupational rhetoric, based on street wisdom and local knowledge. The alternative categorisations constructed by rank-and-file team members to challenge or contextualise expert psychiatric diagnoses are often produced as part of these occupational narratives, and rely on the cultural power of experiential knowledge.

The following extract provides further illustration of the construction of case talk, and shows how information about past contacts can be marshalled as grounds for not accepting a patient as a case. On this occasion the meeting was chaired by the nurse manager.

Extract 3

NM: [reading from referral notes] Saw this patient in clinic on fifteenth March. She was complaining of panic attacks for the last approximately nine months. She puts this down to a marriage which has now ended in divorce and the loss of a pregnancy approximately a year ago. Her two children are disabled. One is mentally handicapped. The other has a kidney problem and is disabled with her leg. Her marriage broke up three years ago. She is now tearful, tends to be rather nasty and does not know what to do. She finds the only way to relax is to take Temazepam medication, during the day. She receives no help from social services at the present time. However, the mental handicap services are involved. She is related to other patients we see. However has little contact with family. Mother died two years ago. Father died a year ago. Past psychiatric history. Brother has treatment.

CPN1: You know whose sister that is? Tom Davies. And what's the other girl, Sandra Hinds?

CPN2: Yeah

CPN1: David Davies is the brother. See that's the sister.

NM: So she is known to you.

CPN1: I think social services have been involved with the daughter, the mentally handicapped daughter.

SW1: Yes, there's definitely some involvement

CPN3: I think the whole family is/

CPN1: Yes screwed up.

SW1: What's her name Pauline?

NM: Pauline James. Yes erm

SW1: She's known to area office.

NM: [looking at notes] Happy, friendly, sad, bothered at present. She's now got an injunction against her husband who came into the house approximately a month ago and started to hit her – her husband at that time and a known drug abuser. Diagnosis at that time was depression with drug abuse. Treatment plan: suggested Prothiaden, Temazepam, two tablets *nocte*. He's going to see her in outpatients in two weeks time. Refer to community mental health team and I would suggest a social worker, preferably a woman involved with this rather difficult case. Erm 29 year old divorced woman who has been depressed and anxious for the last nine months. She has tended to abuse Temazepam and Co-proxamol. However she does have a lot of stress at home with her children and little support. Refer this to the CMHT for support and will see her in outpatients in two weeks time. [five lines identifying GP omitted].

NM: I know you're quite heavy but would you mind taking this on Derek?

SW1: Would I what?

5NM: Would you take this one on?

SW1: What as a case?

NM: Yeah.

SW1: Well, no. I think it's known at the area office. I think it's probably been dealt with. Christine Baker was actually dealing with this at one time.

NM: What's her name?

SW1: Christine Baker, but she's moved on. Somebody... I'm pretty sure somebody in child care or it could be the disabled children, you know, the team. There's a child abuse thing hanging over this and... I think some years ago. That's the kind of case that needs an awful lot of work.

CPN1: Could be that two teams need to be involved though.

SW1: Possibly.

NM: Need to check first to see if she is known then, first of all.

[52 turns omitted, when another patient is discussed before Pauline James' name is reintroduced]

NM Can I just ask again: if I contact John Preece or Gloria Rees at the area office they will be able to tell me if they've this one on their boo//

SW1: Ask if she is currently being seen. She is certainly known.

NM: Okay then.

SW2. I don't know. Rory [psychiatrist] has said she's depressed and anxious.

CPN1: There's a family weakness there really you know.

CPN2: I can remember those in school, very poor.

SW1: They were all very manipulative as well.

CPN2: They were all very poor

CPN3: They've been at outpatients as well.

NM: Like I said she's under... she does have a lot of stress at home with her children and basically needs more support. And it does mention the fact that she receives no help from social services, which I'll chase up. However, the mental handicap services are involved, so I'll see if she is on there.

SW2: With these referrals which are just pumping out asking for support I don't know how much support he thinks we're able to give – ten minutes once a month. I don't know.

CPN3: Well the ongoing ones, I mean they are not going to go away, are they? They'll be added on to//

CPN1: These are time consuming, initially anyway.

SW1: But I don't know how we can take them though. How long can we//

NM: I'll have a chat with him [psychiatrist] tomorrow morning, particularly with the ones that came in this morning.

Here the details of past experience with patients appear to be seen as sufficiently important that the nurse manager is prepared to interrupt his initial case report to seek clarification. In a series of brief turns four different team members indicate that they know the family. Although the information presented is imprecise, and contains at least one self-repair after a mistake (the brother's name), there is a consensus that the family is known to local agencies. Moreover two nurses jointly produce a formulation of the family as defective (CPN3: 'I think the whole family...' CPN1: 'Yes, is screwed up'). The nurse manager finishes the case report and then tries to move directly to allocate the patient to a social worker (a male rather than the female worker requested in the psychiatrist's letter). However, the previous short exchange provides grounds for the social worker (SW1) to do something that is very rare in the taped data: openly to decline to take the case. This is on the basis that the patient is already known to area office. The nurse manager asks for confirmation of the name of the area office social worker handling the case. SW1 is unable to provide firm information but he develops the idea that this is a known case, suggesting that two other specialist teams may be involved, and that there may be 'a child abuse thing hanging over this'. This formulation hints at an unresolved problem and supports his next assertion that it is 'the kind of case that needs an awful lot of work'. CPN1 leaves the way open to take the case by suggesting that two teams may need to be involved, but the nurse manager agrees to check with the area office, 'in the first instance'. In effect the first part of the case discussion ends with an acknowledgement that the case will not be allocated to the team in advance of this enquiry.

The second segment of discussion comes near the end of the session as the nurse manager rehearses the actions he will need to take with a small number of cases that were not allocated. His attempt to get more precise information on which professionals to approach about this patient is unsuccessful. However, any inference that delay in accepting the case, even in the absence of such information, may cause a problem is countered by a series of interjections from other team members, which function to signpost that this is a case for other agencies. This is done by re-framing a case first presented as about an individual woman's 'depression' and 'panic attacks', as a case involving a pathological family. Thus, CPN1 suggests that a 'family weakness' exists, others recount their memories that family members ('they') were 'very poor' or 'manipulative' in school, and that 'they've been at outpatients as well'. Constructing the family as a defective family, with longstanding problems of competence, hints at the unstated possibility of involving the learning disability services. This is picked up by the nurse manager, when he summarises the action he will take by saying that he will 'chase up' social services and also investigate whether the patient is receiving help from 'the mental handicap services'. In the last exchange, the nurse manager moves away from any clear commitment to bring the case back to the team, and agrees to discuss this and other recent referrals with the psychiatrist. The underlying concern with resource constraints surfaces in an early reference to SW1's 'heavy' caseload, and is taken up in the later segment with a chorus of complaints about referrals that are 'just pumping out' from SW2, CPN3, CPN1 and SW1. The nurse manager's promise to talk to the psychiatrist is again linked to the need for better 'gatekeeping', when the team members talk about that day's referrals near the end of the meeting.

Resistance and negotiation

Data such as Extract 3 suggest that patient categorisation and decision outcomes are closely bound up with conflict between the psychiatrist and other team members regarding the proper target group for CMHT work. Challenges by rank-and-file team members to the initial psychiatric categorisations, and the 'referencing work' through which they seek to orient discussions towards a contrasting interpretation of the case, can be seen as resistance to the more inclusive approach to caseloads, aimed at buffering the team from the workload pressures imposed by the psychiatrist (see: Griffiths, 1998). It is therefore instructive to consider what happens in Team B, where staff express similar concerns about workload, but the psychiatrist is present to respond to dissent about the nature of his referrals. Just as happens in the earlier extracts, my data contain many examples where Team B members disagree with an initial psychiatric diagnosis, and seek to put forward a contrasting definition by selectively re-ordering the facts of the case. In Team B, however, such challenges are more likely to lead to protracted negotiations about which version is correct, as in the following example.

Extract 4

CPN1: Oh, yes this is the one we just talked about, Eric Jones. Paul [psychiatrist] saw him. Oh yes, this is the chap with limitations because of physical disability.

SW1: How great is the psychiatric input... problem there Paul?

Psych: He has chronic depressive symptoms and symptoms of anxiety, so I can imagine they need work on. And I think those are in reaction to this physical... I mean, it's a back injury. He currently wears a collar. I think he's in the sick role which is a bit of a... he doesn't like it. The fact that he doesn't like it, that's what generates the depressive bits, the anger. And he turns the anger in on himself. I think he needs, if you like, straightforward counselling, the fact that he isn't limited and looking at the anxiety as well. I mean, he's not severely ill by anybody's//

SW1: Would you think that this is the sort of thing the Adult Services Team would normally deal with?

Psych: No, once you get the sniff of depressive illness they throw it back at us.

SW1: Because they deal all the time with the handicapped, with handicapped adult people, and there must be... You can't say that every person who has been depressed because they're physically ill should be referred to the Psychiatric Team. I mean, they must deal with that element of the condition surely?

SWTL: In theory yes, but in practice it doesn't, for the simple reason, even with child care, if you have a child care problem with depressive illness, they tend to ask us to go and look at it with them. My feelings are: what is the primary handicap? Is it the depressive illnesses or is it the physical problems?

Psych: In terms of primary, there isn't an answer for that, I mean, I think in terms of how it affects his functioning, it's fifty fifty I would guess

In Extract 4, team members use descriptive terms to suggest different underlying categorisations, much as they do in Team A. The psychiatrist seeks to justify his referral. He formulates the patient as someone who, while not 'severely ill', has anxiety symptoms and depression arising from failure to adjust to illness, something that counselling can help correct. The social worker presents depression as a normal response to physical illness, which does not justify specialist psychiatric input. We can describe these different formulations of the patient's condition as competing versions. Acceptance of one version implies acceptance of a particular definition of CMHT work and appropriate service users. In this extract the psychiatrist emphasises the significance of the client's 'chronic depressive symptoms and symptoms of anxiety'. He states that the patient is in the sick role and 'doesn't like it'. According to Parsons' (1951) classic definition, a core element of the sick role is the expectation that patients see illness as an undesirable state and wish to get better, something with which professionals can help. The mention of the anger that the patient turns in on himself, and of the potential use- fulness of counselling, points to a legitimate need for team input. Never- theless, the social worker suggests a referral to the Adult Services Team, a separate interdisciplinary team dealing with adults with physical disabilities. His comment that: 'You can't say that every person who has been depressed because they're physically ill should be referred to the psychiatric team', implicitly suggests the unexceptional, non-pathological character of this case from the psychiatric standpoint. The presence of the psychiatrist, and his sustained defence of his position, makes it harder for others to mount successful challenges to psychiatric categorisations in this team. When the psychiatrist repeats his claim that the client would benefit from counselling, the social worker capitulates, signalling that he accepts the psychiatrist's version of the case by asking for the address of the client so that he can visit him.

The participation of the Team B psychiatrist in meetings made it possible for him to negotiate the eligibility or ineligibility of particular cases, and also to explain general policies. One key difference between the two CMHTs was that the Team B psychiatrist was better able to communicate the desirability of full caseloads in the new market-oriented NHS. His participation in meetings gave him more opportunities to translate the management agenda to the team in ways which acknowledged the problems they were experiencing, represented them as temporary, and emphasised his willingness to share the burdens of this temporary situation. Team A staff were less aware of the pressures felt by their absent psychiatrist/manager, and were more inclined to treat the increased workload as an issue to be dealt with by resisting referrals.

Rank-and-file staff in both CMHTs tend to construct categorisations in the indirect, stepwise way that I have been describing. This resembles Pithouse and Atkinson's (1988) account of social work case talk, in which social workers accomplish 'diagnosis' by means of a narrative/descriptive mode of presentation that makes only sparing use of technical categories. In the supervision meetings recorded for this study, the type of 'problem' under discussion remained largely implicit, so that it was only seen to emerge as fragments of evidence and evaluation were assembled:

> The problem is not specified in terms of a series of traits or propositions: witnessed or suspected faults, peccadillos and clues are selected and emptied out as conversational jigsaw pieces to be arranged and mulled over. The story is constructed by the worker as an act of *bricolage*. That is, bits and pieces of family life are picked out and re-assembled into the narrative format of case talk (Pithouse and Atkinson 1988: 194).

It may plausibly be argued that the discourse of CMHTs represents a meeting and merging of the forms of case talk present in social work and (psychiatric) medicine. While expert psychiatric categorisations have a central place, they are put forward in case discussions that typically involve the narrative/descriptive mode of presentation. The Team B psychiatrist appears to adapt his practice to fit this mode. Although the psychiatrist does sometimes use expert diagnostic labels, these are usually presented as emerging from the team discussion.

Conclusion

Decisions not to allocate resources to referred patients, or to channel them towards less-intensive rather than more-intensive interventions, are forms of rationing central to the work of CMHTs. It has been argued that such decisions emerge from routine case talk, and are closely associated with the implicit as well as the explicit categorisation that occurs in case discussions. The chapter has focused on the nature of these categorisation processes, and particularly on the subtle 'referencing work' through which rank-and-file CMHT members contest definitions and signal the ineligibility of certain referrals as cases. One unfortunate legacy of sociological labelling theory was that it focused attention on the social significance of naming, and diverted attention away from the face-to-face interactions from which 'labels' emerged. Many sociologists still operate with impoverished conceptions of categorisation, in which the emphasis remains on explicit labelling rather than processes of implicit categorisation of the kind described here. This chapter adds to a body of more recent work that aims to develop more sophisticated perspectives on categorisation (see, for example: Snow and Anderson 1987, Ashforth and Humphrey 1995, Crepeau 2000). It suggests that such categorisation processes are closely implicated with selection decisions and have a crucial bearing on patient careers.

Definitional struggles and negotiations about the appropriate target group for CMHT services are a feature of both the teams studied. However, the difference of approach between them lends support to my argument that resource allocation decisions are not just a matter of supply and demand, but also reflect human service workers' subjective understandings of the priorities and pressures affecting them. Rationing decisions, like ethical judgements more generally, have 'tacit components' arising from the unspoken context of professional norms, local knowledge, and assumptions about the constraints affecting routine work (*c.f.* Churchill 1977, Griffiths and Hughes 1998). Thus, it is possible for two CMHTs, serving similar areas but with differing leadership and organisational arrangements, to construct their rules of eligibility in rather different ways. In effect, Team A defined the boundaries of 'serious mental illness' in more restrictive terms than Team B. This resulted in a slower throughput of patients in Team A, than in Team B, with more decisions delayed by requests for further information from referrers. Late in the research period, Team A introduced a waiting list to deal with this 'workload problem', while Team B did not.

One question that merits further investigation is just why so much of the categorisation activity performed by social workers and nurses was implicit rather than explicit. Arguably this reflects the different discursive resources of the various professional disciplines. They have different educational backgrounds and claims to disciplinary knowledge, they are constrained by different chains of accountability, they reach out to different professional and social networks, and they have differing degrees of power to refer, to prescribe, to section and to make other decisions. One reason why social workers and nurses (in CMHTs and elsewhere) favour implicit categorisation over explicit labelling has to do with the category-bound nature of their work: in crude terms doctors diagnose, while social workers and nurses assemble the clinical and social information that will assist in the diagnostic process. In structuring their categorisation activities in the way they do, the participants are paying lip-service (short of full compliance) to the normative requirements of their 'role'. Implicit categorisation can be seen as a less threatening way to question psychiatrists' definitions than open recourse to alternative diagnostic labels. The explanation comes down to a variant of the old distinction between formal and informal social organisation: implicit categorisation is the approach CMHT staff use to get involved in decisions that are not officially within their sphere of work.

If I am right that rationing decisions are closely implicated with the kinds of categorisation processes discussed earlier, this has implications both for policy and for further research. My analysis implies that the rationing of health care emerges from an *ensemble* of micro-level interactions, affected by both intentional and unintentional action, and influenced by a range of contextual/organisational factors. This contrasts with an image of rationing as the product of top-down policies and rational management decisions, whether taken by the UK National Institute of Clinical Excellence or the commissioning manager of a British Primary Care Group. Decisions at those levels are important but they intersect with other powerful influences arising from the tacit backdrop of organisational work, including professional norms, work cultures and understandings of constraints. These things change only slowly and may be partially buffered from top-down political initiatives, such as those recently launched in the UK in the areas of clinical governance and clinical effectiveness. One thing we need to know is just how much 'buffering' occurs. To research the 'real ethics of rationing' (Light 1997: 315), we need studies that get inside the black box of the organisation and shed light on how far 'entrenched institutional, political and professional interests' affect resource allocation at the micro level.

Notes

1   The study was undertaken before the current term 'community mental health nurses' came into usage. Actually 'CPN' seems to have stuck and at the time of writing is still often used by the workers themselves.
2   This is a direct quotation from a meeting in which a social work team leader paraphrases the official guidance.
3   This contrasts with Anspach's (1988) account of medical case presentations, which typically adopt an 'agentless passive voice', and are characterised by de-personalisation, and the use of account markers to distinguish subjective narratives from other parts of the medical report.

References

Anspach, R.R. (1988) Notes on the sociology of medical discourse: the language of case presentation, *Journal of Health and Social Behavior*, 29, 357–75.

Antaki, C. (2001) 'D'you like a drink then do you?' Dissembling language and the construction of an impoverished life, *Journal of Language and Social Psychology*, 20, 196–213.

Ashforth, B.E. and Humphrey, R.H. (1995) Labelling processes in organisations: constructing the individual, *Research in Organisational Behavior*, 17, 413–61.

Audit Commission (1994) *Finding a Place: A Review of Mental Health Services for Adults*. London: The Stationery Office.

Bloor, M. (1976) Bishop Berkeley and the adenotonsillectomy enigma: an exploration of variation in the social construction of medical disposals, *Sociology*, 10, 43–61.

Boden, D. (1994) *The Business of Talk: Organizations in Action*. Cambridge: Polity.

Brown, P. (1989) Psychiatric dirty work revisited: conflicts in servicing non-psychiatric agencies, *Journal of Contemporary Ethnography*, 18, 182–201.

Byrd, D.E. (1981) *Organizational Constraints on Psychiatric Treatment: the Outpatient Clinic*. Greenwich, Connecticut: JAI Press.

Churchill, C.R (1977) Tacit components of medical ethics: making decisions in the clinic, *Journal of Medical Ethics*, 3, 129–32.

Crepeau, E.B. (2000) Reconstructing Gloria: a narrative analysis of team meetings, *Qualitative Health Research*, 10, 766–87.

Department of Health (1994) *Working in Partnership: a Collaborative Approach to Care*. London: The Stationery Office.

Drew, P. (1978) Accusations: the occasioned use of members' knowledge of 'religious geography' in describing events, *Sociology*, 12, 1–22.

Edwards, D. (1991) Categories are for talking, *Theory and Psychology*, 1, 515–42.

Emerson, R.M. (1983) Holistic effects in social control decision making, *Law and Society Review*, 17, 426–55.

Griffiths, L. (1996) *Doing Teamwork: Talk Between Professionals in Community Mental Health Teams*, University of Wales Swansea: Unpublished Ph.D. thesis.

Griffiths, L. (1997) Accomplishing team: teamwork and categorisation in two community mental health teams, *The Sociological Review*, 45, 59–78.

Griffiths, L. (1998) Humour as resistance to professional dominance in community mental health teams. *Sociology of Health and Illness*, 20, 874–95.

Griffiths, L. and Hughes, D. (1993) Typification in a neuro-rehabilitation centre: Scheff revisited? *The Sociological Review*, 41, 415–45.

Griffiths, L. and Hughes, D. (1998) Purchasing in the British NHS: does contracting mean explicit rationing? *Health*, 2, 349–71.

Hak, T. (1998) 'There are clear delusions'. The production of a factual account, *Human Studies*, 21, 419–36.

Heritage, J. and Lindstrom, A. (1998) Motherhood, medicine, and morality: scenes from a medical encounter, *Research on Language and Social Interaction*, 31, 397–438.

Hester, S. (1992) Recognising references to deviance in referral talk. In Watson, G and Seiler, R.M. (eds) *Text in Context: Contributions to Ethnomethodology*. Newbury Park: Sage.

Hughes, D. (1976) 'Everyday and medical knowledge in categorizing patients'. In Dingwall, R., Heath, C., Reid, M. and Stacey, M. (eds.) *Health Care and Health Knowledge*. London: Croom Helm.

Hughes, D. (1980) The ambulance journey as an information generating process, *Sociology of Health and Illness*, 2, 115–32.

Hughes, D. and Griffiths, L. (1996) "But if you look at the coronary anatomy...": risk and rationing in cardiac surgery, *Sociology of Health and Illness*, 18, 172–97.

Jayyusi, L. (1984) *Categorization and the Moral Order*. London: Routledge and Kegan Paul.

Jeffery, R. (1979) Normal rubbish: deviant patients in casualty departments. *Sociology of Health and Illness*, 1, 90–107.

Kelly, M. and May, D. (1982) Good and bad patients: a review of the literature and a theoretical critique, *Journal of Advanced Nursing*, 7, 147–56.

Light, D. (1997) The real ethics of rationing, *British Medical Journal*, 315, 112–15.

Murcott, A. (1981), 'On the typification of "bad patients"'. In Atkinson, P. and Heath, C.C. (eds) *Medical Work: Realities and Routines*. Farnborough: Gower.

Parsons, T. (1951) *The Social System*. New York: The Free Press of Glencoe.

Pithouse, A. and Atkinson, P. (1988) Telling the case: occupational narrative in a social work office. In Coupland, N. (ed) *Styles of Discourse*. London: Croom Helm.

Poirer, S. and Brauner, D.J. (1988) Ethics and the daily language of medical discourse, *Hastings Centre Report*, August/September, 5–9.

Sacks, H. (1972a) An initial investigation of the usability of conversational data for doing sociology. In Sudnow, D. (ed) *Studies in Social Interaction*. New York: Free Press.

Sacks, H. (1972b) On the analyzability of stories by children. In Gumperz, J.J. and Hymes, D. (eds) *Directions of Sociolinguistics*. New York: Holt, Rinehart and Winston.

Scheff, T.J., (1965) Typification in the diagnostic practices of rehabilitation agencies. In Sussman, M.B. (ed) *Sociology and Rehabilitation*. Washington D.C.: A.S.A.

Shears, M. and Coleman, M. (1999) Mental health nursing policy: an exploratory qualitative study of managers' opinions, *Journal of Advanced Nursing*, 29, 1385–92.

Shepherd, G. (1995) Commentary. Finding a place: a review of mental health services for adults, *Journal of Mental Health*, 4, 9–16.

Snow, D.A. and Anderson, L. (1987) Identity work among the homeless: the verbal construction and avowal of personal identities, *American Journal of Sociology*, 92, 1336–71.

Tredget, J. and Bowler, N. (2000) Divided priorities: mental health referrals, *Nursing Times*, 96, 47–8.

Watson, R. (1976) Some conceptual issues in the social identification of victims and offenders. In Viano, E. (ed) *Victims and Society*. Washington, D.C.: Vintage.

8

Subverting criteria: the role of precedent in decisions to finance surgery

John Heritage, Elizabeth Boyd and Lawrence Kleinman

Introduction

In their classic description of the acculturation of medical students into the ways of medical practice, Becker *et al.* (1961) noted the central position of clinical experience in medical decision making. Based on the physician's personal, firsthand experience in observing, diagnosing, and treating patients, clinical experience was seen as both fundamental and necessary for any competent physician. Indeed, clinical experience was understood to be preferable to abstract scientific evidence or 'book learning' as a basis for clinical judgment. As Becker *et al.* wrote:

> Clinical experience ... gives the doctor the knowledge he needs to treat patients successfully, even though that knowledge has not yet been systematized and scientifically verified. One does not acquire this knowledge through academic study but by seeing clinical phenomena and dealing with clinical problems first hand. Clinical experience, even though it substitutes for scientifically verified knowledge, can be used to legitimate a choice of procedures for a patient's treatment and can even be used to rule out use of some procedures which have been scientifically established (1961: 231).

In the 40 years since Becker and his colleagues wrote, there have been repeated efforts to systematise medical decision making and reduce the amount of variation in the diagnosis and treatment of patients (Berg 1997). From standard practice guidelines and computer-based protocols to decision analysis and evidence-based medicine, each effort to systematise medical decision making is ultimately designed to address concerns that clinical experience alone is insufficient as a basis for diagnosis and treatment decisions; a more rational, evidence-based system is also necessary (Berg 1997).

Despite these consistent efforts by a variety of institutions, including clinical societies, third-party payers, and government agencies, many physicians continue to substitute clinical experience even when it contrasts with scientific knowledge. This chapter examines the pervasiveness of appeals to clinical experience in the context of utilisation review, one recent effort to systematise and rationalise medical decision making in the United States. Specifically, we focus on the use of precedent, meaning by this the belief that because one has used a procedure in the past with a particular patient, one is justified in using the same procedure again for the same patient in a similar condition. In this use of precedent, the fact that the patient's condition justified a procedure in the past is treated as a transparent argument for a similar claim in the present. Thus, buoyed by precedent, the past use of a procedure can serve as a self-evident *justification* for its use in the future. This notion of precedent may lie at the heart of various 'medical myths' – practices or procedures that are maintained, and often promoted, even though they have no basis in the scientific literature.

In this chapter, we focus on a commitment to a medical precedent that appears to be entrenched in the culture of otolaryngologists: the belief that prior tympanostomy surgery warrants subsequent tympanostomy surgery in the same patient, even in the absence of evidence to support such a conclusion. We examine the presence and functioning of this belief in the context of prospective utilisation review – a bureaucratic process in which attending physicians must justify the need for tympanostomy surgery to the medical representatives of insurance companies. Prospective utilisation review (UR) is an attempt to restrict treatments to patients who are most likely to benefit from them, and to minimise the use of inappropriate procedures which waste resources and represent poor quality health care. In our data, prospective UR involves the implementation of explicit criteria which must be met to approve cases for surgery. This is a context in which justifications for surgeries, including the use of precedent, are densely present.

Our chapter begins with a description of the review process, the medical condition, otitis media, for which tympanostomy tube insertion was proposed, and the data on which our analysis is based. We then examine the ways that an orientation to prior surgeries permeates the review process, and, finally, we consider how the myth of prior surgery may provide for accountability in the context of the review.

Prospective utilisation review and the process of rationalising decisions

Utilisation review is one method by which third-party payers can control health care costs either by requiring physicians to try alternative, less expensive treatments first or, as in this case, by attempting to limit the use of medical procedures or technologies to those clinical circumstances for which they are most likely to be effective, based on current knowledge and expert belief. The UR firm we studied was a national firm that contracted with various third-party payers to conduct prospective utilisation reviews for a variety of surgical procedures, including tympanostomy, tonsillectomy, arthroscopy, haemorrhoidectomy, hysterectomy, and carpal tunnel surgery. The UR firm convened panels of clinical and academic experts to develop explicit criteria to be used to determine the appropriateness or medical necessity of the proposed procedure. In this UR firm, appropriateness was defined as situations in which the expected health benefits would exceed the expected negative health consequences by a sufficiently wide margin (Kleinman *et al.* 1994, Kleinman *et al.* 1997). The reviews were *prospective*: cases that failed to meet the criteria were not covered by the third-party payer and the surgery was not likely to be performed.

The UR firm used a two-step process to evaluate proposed surgeries. In the first-level review, a nurse-reviewer conducted a telephone interview with a member of the attending surgeon's (ENT/otolaryngologist's) office staff who read from the patients written chart. These interviews were guided by an interactive computer programme, using a smart logic branching algorithm, designed such that each answer to a question prompted another question until a 'threshold' was reached and the case was approved for surgery.

Cases that were not approved for surgery at this level, approximately 30 per cent of the cases in the time period we examined, were forwarded to the second-level review in which a physician-reviewer interviewed the attending physician by telephone. The purpose of the second-level review was to determine the existence of any new information (that was not contained in the written record) or any extenuating circumstances that would override the criteria (such as the presence of certain conditions that were not included in the first-level review protocol, *e.g.*, Down's syndrome or cleft palate). At this time, the physician-reviewer had available for consultation the 'paper trail' from the first-level review – a computer-generated listing of the protocol (interview) results; a list of the criteria necessary to approve the case; and any additional summary handwritten notes from the nurse-reviewer. Thus, in each instance, the reviewer had the data in advance of the interview to know which aspects of the case were sufficiently problematic for the case to fail the first-level review.

During the review, the reviewer's tasks, as defined by the UR firm, were to verify the accuracy and completeness of the information gathered in the first-level review, to identify and assess the *criterial* relevance of any new information offered by the surgeon, and to identify and evaluate any potentially extenuating circumstances that might bear on the appropriateness of the surgery. On the basis of any new or additional information, the reviewer either overturned the first-level review and recommended the case for surgery or sustained the first-level review and did not recommend the case for surgery. Cases not recommended were eligible for appeal[1].

Otitis media and its treatment

All the cases under review in this study involved patients who suffered from otitis media, a condition characterised by the build-up of fluid or the development of infection in the middle ear. Otitis media is the most commonly diagnosed ailment in children, affecting some two-thirds of American children by the age of two and accounting for more than 14 per cent of all visits to the paediatrician, and more than 20 per cent of all visits to the otolaryngologist (Kleinman et al. 1994).

Otitis media generally takes two forms: acute otitis media (AOM) and otitis media with effusion (OME). Acute otitis media involves active infection, and generally includes symptoms such as fussiness, pain or fever. It generally resolves after a course of antibiotic therapy, but may frequently recur (Bluestone and Klein 1988; Kleinman et al. 1994). Otitis media with effusion (also known as 'serous' or 'secretory' otitis media (SOM)) involves the presence of fluid in the middle ear but the ear itself is not inflamed and there is no active infection. OME may arise spontaneously, or as a sequela of AOM. It may lead to fussiness or temporary hearing loss, but is frequently asymptomatic. OME frequently resolves spontaneously or with a single course of antibiotic therapy.

Although young children are especially vulnerable to middle ear infections because of anatomical immaturity, otitis media is not generally considered a serious health threat. AOM's main symptoms, fever and/or pain in the ear, can cause distress in young children, but in most cases do not represent a serious hazard. There are a few very infrequent suppurative complications of otitis media, which may result in permanent hearing loss. Temporary hearing loss commonly occurs during the period when fluid is in the middle ear: controversy exists as to whether this is associated with significant delays in language development. The natural history of otitis media is that the severity and frequency of illness moderates with increasing age.

An alternative treatment to antibiotic therapy is the surgical insertion of tympanostomy, or pressure equalisation (PE) tubes (also known as grommets). These are small plastic or metal prosthetic devices that are inserted into the ear to help manage persistent effusion or recurrent infections. PE tubes function by assisting the Eustachian tube to maintain equal pressure on both sides of the ear drum (Bluestone and Klein 1988). At the time of insertion, fluid or accumulated material is usually drained by the surgeon. The insertion of PE tubes for otitis media is extremely common, with some 670,000 surgeries conducted in 1988 in the US, making it the most common operation for children (Kleinman et al. 1994). Typically, PE tubes will remain in the ear for a period of up to two years. Though they are normally extruded spontaneously, surgical removal is occasionally necessary. The annual cost of tympanostomy tube surgery to the US health care system exceeds one billion dollars annually (Cantekin *et al.* 1991).

Despite their pervasive use, however, the benefits of PE tubes are uncertain. According to some researchers, antibiotic treatment is equally effective in managing otitis media and is both less costly and less risky than surgery[2][3]. For this reason, as an overall strategy of cost containment, some health plans now require certain standards of prior treatment, such as a course of antibiotics or watchful waiting, before reimbursement for tympanostomy surgery[4]. The UR firm in this study implements such requirements for third-party payers, requiring otolaryngologists to meet certain criteria (involving clinical and treatment history) before reimbursement. Gathering information regarding prior treatment and clinical symptoms constitutes the focus of the utilisation review described here.

The data

The data for this study come from a stratified random sample of 108 audiotaped reviews, conducted by telephone, between 13 physician-reviewers and 108 specialists (10 primary care physicians and 98 otolaryngologists). The physician-reviewers, representing a California-based, national utilisation review (UR) firm, were board-certified specialists in either otolaryngology, paediatrics, or internal medicine. All were licensed to practice medicine in the state of California.

The attending physicians under review had proposed the surgical insertion of tympanostomy tubes for the management of recurrent acute otitis media or otitis media with effusion. The physicians were located throughout the country. The audio recordings were made as part of the record-keeping routine of the UR firm, and all the doctors were aware of the recording. Patients agree to prospective or retrospective review as a part of their personal insurance contracts. The tape recorder was under the control of the reviewer and was, in most instances, switched on as contact with the doctor was established. Names and identifying characteristics of the physician-reviewers, the attending physicians under review, and the patients have been changed.

This sample was drawn from a total population of 5214 tympanostomy cases reviewed by the UR firm between 1 April, 1990 and 31 July, 1991 for three national third-party payer organisations (*i.e.* health care insurance companies) covering some 5.6 million Americans. Of these 5214 reviewed cases, 1448 (or 28 per cent) were found to be inappropriate after a first-step review (described below). Of these cases, 942 were reviewed by physician-reviewers who were employed by the UR firm. These 942 cases form the core sample from which the calls analysed in this study were drawn. The sample was stratified by type of appeal available and relative volume of cases handled by each reviewer. Low-volume reviewers were over-sampled to increase reviewer variability. The sample was also stratified by outcome or decision, with 71 cases approved for surgery, 31 cases denied, and six cases decision-deferred pending confirmation of history from the referring physician. For this chapter, 12 cases were eliminated from the sample, 6 which had no decision (or decision pending) and 6 with incomplete records.

The average length of a review was approximately four minutes. The shortest call lasted about one minute; the longest stretched to 12 minutes.

The criteria

The criteria used by the reviewers in determining the appropriateness of surgery were developed by the UR firm, based on the recommendations of a panel of national experts (5 paediatricians and four otolaryngologists). This panel synthesised the current literature on the medical management of otitis media, in order to develop a set of evidence-based explicit criteria for tympanostomy. Using the two-round modified Delphi process developed by Brook et al. (1986), 80 specific clinical scenarios were evaluated as potential indications for surgery, and were rated on a nine-point ordinal scale with the following interpretation, 1–3 inappropriate, 4–6 equivocal or uncertain, and 7–9, appropriate. The criteria were to be applied to those clinical findings that could be documented by the physician or by the medical record.

The reviewers were mandated to be oriented by these criteria as they made determinations regarding the appropriateness of surgery. The attending physician under review consulted the patient's clinical record, as needed, to answer the reviewer's questions about symptoms, diagnosis, and treatment. Factors such as the age of the child, the presence of fluid in the ear (effusion) and its duration, amount of hearing loss, the frequency of AOM, type of antibiotic treatments, the presence of learning or developmental difficulties, and exceptional circumstances (such as cleft palate or Down's Syndrome) were possible indications for surgery.

These criteria combine in a variety of ways. For example, otitis media with effusion [OME] involves a combination of some 64 indications. Age is the first indication: patients under age three were subject to different criteria than were patients over age three. Duration of effusion (how long the patient had fluid in the ear) is the second indication – any duration less than 60 days, regardless of other factors, would be found inappropriate. Marked otoscopic findings (upon physical examination, whether the middle ear shows retraction pockets and/or the absence of air bubbles) was the next indication, followed by a hearing loss of at least 25 db (as measured by an audiogram) and a trial course of antibiotics (of at least 10 days). Complications of otitis media were a further set of indications, and included acute mastoiditis, facial palsy, meningitis, and brain abscess. Table 1 shows a range of values of indicators for otitis media with effusion, and the guidelines for their evaluation in relation to surgery.

For example, as shown in Table 1, a patient over the age of three, with a history of otitis media for 120 days, mild otoscopic findings, and a trial course of antibiotics would be approved for surgery; while a patient under three, with mild otoscopic findings, with a history of more than 120 days of effusion, and no antibiotics would not be approved. A patient over the age of three, who has had an effusion of 95 days, a normal hearing test, and a trial of antibiotics would be approved for surgery; a child over three, who has had 120 days of effusion, a hearing loss of 25 db, but no antibiotics would not be approved. A child with acute mastoiditis, meningitis or brain abscess would be approved regardless of other indications, as would a child

Table 1: *Criteria for assessing the appropriateness of tympanostomy tube insertion for otitis media with persistent effusion with mild* otoscopic findings*

	Duration of otitis media with effusion, days			
	< 60	*60–90*	*91-120*	*> 120*
Appropriate for Surgery?				
Mild otoscopic findings				
No hearing test/age < 3 No course of antibiotics	No	No	No	No
No hearing test/age < 3 One or more courses of antibiotics	No	No	Equivocal	Equivocal
No hearing test/age ≥ 3 No course of antibiotics	No	No	No	No
No hearing test/age ≥ 3 One or more courses of antibiotics	No	No	Equivocal	Equivocal
Normal hearing test No course of antibiotics	No	No	No	No
Normal hearing test One or more courses of antibiotics	No	No	Equivocal	Equivocal
Abnormal hearing test No course of antibiotics	No	No	No	No
Abnormal hearing test One or more courses of antibiotics	No	Equivocal	Equivocal	Yes

* Mild otoscopic findings are present when no posterior superior retraction pockets are noted and/or the eardrum is not densely impacted.

The UR firm recommends in favour of surgery when the appropriateness rating is 'yes' or 'equivocal'.

with Down's Syndrome or cleft palate. These last patient characteristics were not included in the algorithm, but were considered extenuating circumstances that should overturn the first-level decision upon their discovery by the reviewer. It should be noted that, consistent with the medical literature, the expert panel did not include a prior history of treatment with tympanostomy tubes as relevant to assessing the appropriateness of current proposals for surgery.

The outcome of the review process is the reviewer's recommendation to the insurance company as to whether tympanostomy tubes are appropriate for this patient at this time. The recommendation either supports the conclusions of the first-level review that the case is inappropriate, or overturns it. Although reviewers neither approve nor deny care directly, for the sake of clarity we use these terms to describe their recommendations. These recommendations, which are frequently described in these terms by the reviewers themselves, are normally conveyed to the attending physician at the end of the phone call.

Rationalisation versus precedent

As one strategy for controlling the costs of health care, the reviews examined here represent an incursion into the previously unregulated area of clinical judgment. They represent an effort to rationalise decision making about tympanostomy tube surgery by means of explicit criteria which the reviewers have contracted to implement. However, despite the fact that outcomes should strongly correlate with the explicit criteria, they do not. While the reviewers never recommended against surgery that the criteria would support as appropriate, they frequently approved surgeries that the criteria would have denied. Of the 66 cases in our data set that they approved for surgery, 47 (71 per cent) did not meet the UR firm's criteria (Kleinman et al. 1997: 499). Table 2 uses logistic regression to model the major factors predicting the reviewers' decisions to overturn the negative first-level review and approve the case for surgery.

Table 2 demonstrates that a history of previous tympanostomy tube surgery is strongly associated with a reviewer's recommendation in favour of surgery, even when controlling for the level of appropriateness. To examine this finding in more detail, we turned to the written records that summarised each review, and to audiotapes of the second-level reviews themselves.

The recorded data

We collected detailed data on 96 cases. The data included:

1. The print out from the computer-guided first-level review between the nurse-reviewer and the ENT's office staff. Included with the print out

Table 2: *Factors impacting positive reviewer recommendations for surgery*

Variable	Odds ratio	95% Confidence interval	p
Age	1.03	0.78–1.36	.83*
Appropriateness rating	4.55	2.02–10.25	< .001*
Female sex	8.15	1.23–53.84	.03
Clinical severity†	1.02	1.00–1.03	.01*
Excess duration††	1.95	1.06–3.58	.03
History of prior tubes	30.94	2.43–394.81	.01

* These three variables have a defined relationship with the criteria and are included in this model only for the purposes of controlling for confounding while evaluating the other three variables.

† Clinical severity represents an interaction between the duration of effusion and the frequency of acute otitis media.

†† Excess duration represents, in 30-day intervals, the length of time that an effusion was asserted to have been present in excess of the documented duration of the effusion. This variable is included as a marker for the effect of undocumented clinical assertions on the outcome of the review.

Source: Kleinman *et al.* (1997) 'Adherence to prescribed explicit criteria during utilization review of tympanostomy: an analysis of communications between attending and reviewing physicians', *Journal of the American Medical Association* (1997) 278, 6, 497–501.

were handwritten notes which the nurse-reviewer made on a scratchpad and incorporated into the case record;

2. Tape recordings of the second-level telephone reviews between the UR firm's reviewers and the attending ENTs (surgeons), in which a decision regarding the medical necessity of the proposed surgery was reached;

3. The notes the physician-reviewers made justifying their recommendations made at the conclusion of their calls.

Results

Of the 96 cases examined, 44 per cent (42/96) of the patients had previously had tympanostomy surgery and 83 per cent (35/42) of these were approved for additional surgery. As Table 3 shows, references to these patients' prior surgeries surfaced at every point in the review process, despite the fact that the criteria for approval did not include prior surgery.

It is noteworthy that references to prior surgeries emerged both in the written records produced by the nurses performing the first-level review, and in the reviewers' notes on the second-level reviews. Discussion of prior surgeries were also an extensive and lively feature of the telephone reviews themselves, and emerged both in the clinical history of the case, and in the final section of the discussion between the reviewer and the attending physician during which the reviewers announced their recommendations and described the rationales for them.

Table 3: *Where were previous PE tubes mentioned*

Nurse 1st level review scratchpad*	32/96 (33.3%)
During the clinical discussion**	41/96 (42.7%)
As part of the verbal decision rationale	10/96 (10.4%)
Physician 2nd level review notes justifying the final decision	33/96 (34.4%)
Total number of cases in which there has been previous surgery***	42/96 (46.9%)
Total number of reviews	96

* Does not include three cases in which the nurse notes indicate that surgery had previously been approved, but not performed.
** Includes three cases in which the reviewer asked about prior tympanostomy surgery, and found that there had been none.
*** Based on written records associated with these cases, and the review telephone conversations.

During the first level review:
Evidence for the significance of a prior history of tympanostomy tube surgery in the clinical culture we studied initially emerges in the first-level review. Although we do not have recordings of these conversations, we do have the results of the computer-assisted interview together with the nurse's 'scratchpad' notes. The scratchpad provides an opportunity for the reviewing nurses to note factors that they or the attending physician's office staff consider important, or which they think the reviewers will find relevant, and which are not addressable directly through the computer-assisted portion of the interview. The nurses made scratchpad entries documenting prior surgery in 32 of the 42 cases in which prior surgery had occurred, or just over three-quarters of them.

Typically, these observations were unstressed and embedded in a general narrative of the patient's condition, as in (1):

1. Nurse scratchpad notes (Case #1949)

Dx: Middle ear infection
Hx: Tubes inserted 11/28/89
       Seen in MDO 03/21/90 Tubes dry
PE   09/07/90 tympanic membrane dull. Right tube out
       O hearing test done
       No documentation as to when tube fell out
       No otitis media documented since last November.

In other cases, however, the summary was more emphatic in its representation of previous PE tube treatment, as in (2):

2. Nurse scratchpad notes (Case #1149)

DX: OM with effusion
       This will be the patient's third set of tubes

8/21/90 (L) OM with effusion, wick placed. Patient was placed on Ceclor
10/90 (R) ear ok, (L) som placed on ceclor
11/90 Both ears were clear
3/25/91 mother called: patient has bilateral ear pain without fever
3/27/91 child was seen dx: OM with effusion
Last hearing test 11/90.

While the notes in (2) appear to suggest the role of antibiotics in clearing the patient's condition, others imply a more significant role for the previous PE tubes, as in (3) and (4):

3. Nurse scratchpad notes (Case #4650)

DX: (R) middle ear infection
Patient has had previous tubes
Last tubes were placed 11/88
4/90 (R) tube was blocked
6/90 Ears were clear and the patient was doing well
10/90 (R) tube was out and effusion was present, tympanogram was flat and mild conductive hearing loss was present on the (R)
Hearing on the (L) was normal

4. Nurse scratchpad notes (Case #9064)

Dx: Chronic left SOM
Hx: June 1989: bilat. titanium tubes placed.
May '90: Left tube extruded. June '90 Left SOM, wick placed
July '90: right tube in place, ear dry. Ear gtts in left.
Pt. to be checked in 6 mos. Oct '90 Pt on Augmentin for OM
Jan '91: Pt. on Extendryl and doing Valsalva
Feb '91: Left drum retracted. Hearing loss of 40–60 db in left ear.
Plan: To replace left titanium tube

In (3) and (4), improvements and deteriorations in the patient's condition are more closely associated, at least by implication, with the presence or absence of tubes.

In addition, the nurses also entered a small additional number of *negative observations* into the scratchpad: that is, observations that the child had *not* had previous tube surgery, or that s/he had been scheduled for surgery, but that the surgery had not been carried out. The fact that nurses chose to record these negative observations speak to their lively significance for the nurses, or at least for their perceptions that this history would be relevant for the physician-reviewers who would be following up denied cases with a second level review. Although the criteria for approving surgeries were designed to exclude prior surgery as a feature of decision-making, the presence or absence of prior surgeries retained a real relevance for the participants at this lowest tier of decision-making in utilisation review.

Finally, in a majority of cases (59 per cent), the nurses' scratchpad entries were followed up with some reviewer-initiated inquiry about the prior surgeries, most commonly at the very beginning of the review process. Thus, the prior surgery was not only considered to be *relevant* to a case by a nurse-reviewer, it also became *consequential* as shaping the content of the second level reviews.

During the second level reviews:
Since prior surgery was not one of the criteria on which the reviewer was instructed to evaluate a patient's case, it might be expected that the nurse-reviewer's notes documenting such surgery would not enter into the second-level, physician-physician review. However, our findings are consistent with the alternative that prior surgery is an important feature of the shared understanding between the reviewing physician and the attending physician. Prior surgeries appeared as a topic in 41 (or 43 per cent) of our review conversations. In two-thirds of these cases, the prior surgery was introduced at the very beginning of the review, establishing it as a significant (*i.e.* mentionable) part of the patient's clinical history. In some instances, the prior surgery was mentioned by the reviewer as the very first element of the patient's background, as in (5),

---

Rev = Physician reviewing the case for the UR firm
Att = Attending physician (normally the surgeon proposing the surgery).

---

5. [9064]   [Reviewer shows knowledge of prior surgery]
```
 1 Rev:     ..... I appreciate your calling us ba:ck
 2          .hh U::h (.) I'm with a physician group doing
 3          preauthorization for the (NAME)'s insurance
 4          company: (.) an:d you may hear a beep as we
 5       →  routinely record. .h[h Uh I know she's ha:d u:h PE
 6 Att:                         ['ka:y,
 7 Rev:  →  tu:bes befo:re (.) some titanium tu:bes an' then
 8       →  (.) one of 'em is ou:t h .hh (.) and she was infec-
 9          infected back I think in u:h .hh in u:h (      )
10          at least a (wick) was placed. = I guess it- the right
11          tube maybe was infected and then .hh and she's got
12          a large hearing lo:ss like forty decibels. h [.hh U:m
13 Att:                                                  [Yeah.
14 Rev:     (.) is she:: uh- th'- th'- question that came up
15          on 'er is whether she's been: (.) treated medically
16          with antibiotics t' try t' c- c- eh cu:re the:: curren:t
```

```
17              eh serous otitis medi[a on the left with antibiotics.
18 Att:                         [No no.  She doesn't have- she
19              doesn't have serous otitu- .h[h She has adhesive otitis.
20 Rev:                         [Oh.
```

In this instance, the reviewer begins his consideration of the case at hand by reviewing the information that he already knows about the patient. Although the first item on the computer-generated printout from which the patient's medical history is available is the patient's age, which is the first decision branch in the criteria's algorithm, the reviewer begins the history with a description of the patient's previous tympanostomy tube insertion, which was the first item noted in the nurse's scratchpad notes (lines 5–8). Indeed the reviewer's opening remarks follow the nurse's scratchpad notes in (4) very closely. In this case, as in others, it is virtually certain that the reviewer focused on the nurse's summary scratchpad notes as narrative guidance for the case, rather than the more complex and less accessible computer-generated paper trail.

In this context, the reviewer's first mention of criteria-relevant information does not come until line 12 (the 40-decibel hearing loss) and his question concerning antibiotic treatment, at lines 14–17, displays the problematic aspect of the case vis-a-vis the criteria: the patient had apparently not been treated with antibiotics. Despite this, the reviewer's first characterisation of the patient had to do with her prior tubes.

Similarly, in (6), the reviewer mentions the patient's prior surgery near the beginning of his review of her history, second only to her apparent cleft lip repair, a circumstance that might be evaluated as extenuating and therefore overriding the criteria[5].

```
6. [4687]   [Reviewer shows knowledge of prior surgery]
 1 Rev:    I'm doing a preauthorisation for the [NAME]
 2         insurance [h company an::' I appreciate your ti:me, =
 3 Att:              [Uh huh,
 4 Rev:    [=you may hear a bee:p as we: (.) routinely record
 5 Att:    [Sure, no problem,
 6 Rev:    .hh[hh I kno:w uh the child has a- (uh) had a cleft
 7 Att:        [Sure,
 8 Rev:  → repa::ir: i[n February and PE tubes were pla:c[ed and
 9 Att:             [Uh huh,                          [Right.
10 Rev:  → now .hhh and now they're ou:t. .hhh U:h do you know
11         anything about the past history? Has the kid had a
12         lotta trouble prior to tha:t with: u:h needing PE tu:bes?
13 Att:    U::m I think this has only been his first se:t?
14 Rev:    Mmhm.
15 Att:    But you kno- uh- you kno:w with ˙(a)˙ cleft palate an' all
16         [that stuff-
```

```
17 Rev:    [We:ll, yeah, in fact- uh I'm an otalaryngologist and
18         cleft pa:late that's tru:e, = (if) you're cleft lip I'm not su:re
19         that it's the: automatic thi:ng but it-
```

In this instance, the reviewer begins his review of the case by mentioning the facts of the history that he does know: that the patient had had cleft repair and prior tubes. As in (5), this was raised as a topic even before the patient's age (which, in this case, later became the most relevant aspect of the patient's history – the child was less than a year old, which the reviewer treated as a complicating factor in making his decision). As both (5) and (6) show, the reviewers treated the patients' prior history of tympanostomy tube insertion to be not only relevant to the case, but *immediately* relevant, as evidenced by its mention at the start of the review.

This pattern of early establishment of a patient's history of prior tubes held across cases, even when the reviewer did not already know that the patient had had such surgery, as in (7) and (8).

```
7. [1231]   [Rev queries prior surgery]
 1 Rev:    Alright the i:nformation I have is she is about two::
 2         and a half¿
 3 Att:    Yes,
 4 Rev:    And pt .hh she:'s had uh:: ear infe:ctions in the
 5         past¿ Ah:: although I don't have too much information
 6         on (.) how many in the last six months let say .hhh
 7    →    ah::: I don't know if she's had tubes befo:re¿ (.)
 8         Actually I don't have too much i(h)n(h)formation on her
 9         maybe you could uh te:ll me a[bout that,
10 Att:                                 [I uh:: I don't think she has
11         tubes befo:re,
12 Rev:    Oka::y,
13 Att:    An:d according to the mo:ther she has repeated
14         ear infections she was treated with amoxicillin and
15         (she      ) .hhh and still she is complaining of the
16         ears pulling in the ears and she is not hearing as
17         good as she should¿

8. [6896]   [Rev queries prior surgery]
 1 Rev:    Ye:s. Let me inform < you you';ll hear a beep in th' >
 2         ba:ckground, = That's part of the recording.
 3 Att:    A:lright,
 4 Rev:    (h)O:ka::y, hh And you were gonna say abou::t uh
 5         (Mary), (.) .hhh
 6 Att:    'ea uh- she uh- (.) we're gonna put- we were gonna
 7         pla:n on puttin' tu:bes in 'er ears. =
 8 Rev: →  = Uh hu::h, has she had tubes before?
 9 Att:    'et's see. I think she ha:s.
```

```
10 Rev:    Mm[hm,
11 Att:        [U::m (0.4) lemme just look here. (0.2) .h Yeah she
12         ha:d 'em once befo:re (0.2) i:n March of eighty seven.
13 Rev:    Mmhm.
```

In both (7) and (8), the reviewers again raise prior tubes as a relevant topic, although in these instances, that fact remains to be established as the reviewers did not know that aspect of the patients' histories. The posing of a question to the surgeon regarding prior surgery explicitly raises the surgery as a relevant topic for the review, again, even though it is not relevant to the criteria (and is not considered an extenuating circumstance).

The establishment of prior surgery as a relevant aspect of the patient's history is, on one hand, perhaps not surprising – for those patients who had had the surgery, it was undeniably part of their medical history. Moreover, it may be that the reviewers treated the fact of prior surgery as an indicator of possible extenuating circumstances that would emerge in the subsequent discussion of the topic. However these references to prior surgery also embody an understanding, shared between the reviewer and the attending physician, that prior surgery is a relevant consideration in evaluating cases for surgery – a medical myth unsupported in the scientific literature.

It is striking that the topic of prior surgery was regularly introduced at the start of the review – the reviewer either mentioned his/her knowledge of it or s/he inquired into it at the beginning of the review of the patient's history. Thus, from the outset, that aspect of the patient's past was established. Moreover, prior surgery was regularly mentioned before any of the criteria-relevant aspects of the case, and, especially, before those aspects that worked against approving the case were mentioned. Analysis of the tape recordings of the reviews suggests that this placement of the topic of prior surgery early in the conversation is significant for the resources it seems to provide.

First, it topicalises a matter which, from the perspective of the attending physician, would be grounds for approving the case. By inviting conversation about a factor which is favourable to surgery, it establishes a collegial stance (Boyd 1998) towards the attending physician, and may suggest that the reviewer is not prejudiced against the possibility of surgery. Second, the introduction of the patient's prior surgery puts in place a possible resource that each participant may later make use of. The previous surgeries may be invoked by the attending physician, whether immediately or distally, to justify the current proposal for surgery. Given the acknowledgement of its significance embodied in the reviewer's attention to the matter, the case may become more difficult to deny. It may also be a resource for the reviewer, helping to establish the seeds of an account for his/her decision, even before that decision has been reached. This is particularly significant in the context of reviews that involve conflict, and in which the reviewer may ultimately prefer to have a consensual, but inappropriate, basis on which to approve a case and avoid an emotionally draining disagreement with a peer (Boyd 1997).

The explicit orientation of the reviewer and the surgeon to prior surgery as a relevant account for proposing surgery is commonplace in these inter- actions. In cases where the reviewer did not reference prior surgery, the attending physicians' narratives described prior surgeries and their sequelae as part of building a case for their decisions to propose surgery. Most com- monly (nine of 16 cases), they mentioned previous surgeries as the first component of a response to a request for medical information about the patient. In many of these cases, this information was explicitly introduced as a justification for the current proposal for surgery, as in (9) and (10) below:

9. [8131]   [Attending physician immediately cites prior surgery]
```
 1 Att:    Have y- Has the nurses eh- eh- e::h- in your- c- eh-
 2         done- d- dealing with your computer not given you the
 3         information?
 4 Rev:    Oh. They did. But you know the:- whatever they give me
 5         is (.) e- effusion which is only four weeks o [::ld
 6 Att:  →                                              [(Do you)
 7         kno:w that this child has had tubes on two previous
 8         occasions?
 9 Rev:    .h Well, e::h,    ((pages turning))
10         (0.2)
11 Att:  → Do you know that?
12 Rev:    No- Y'know I- I appreciate if you give me your information
13         [an'
14 Att:    [The- the child has had t- eh tubes on two previous
15         occasions. < Has also undergone a T an' A for this problem
16         ₀hh The child continues to have effusions (.) now that
17       → the tubes have extruded.
```

In this case the attending physician's rather hectoring initial response to the reviewer's request for information about the effusion treats the child's previous surgical history as self-evidently relevant to the present review, and this is subsequently underscored by his explicit linkage (lines 16–17) between the current effusion and the now extruded tubes. And in (10), the attending physician's initial reference to previous tubes is connected to the child's present condition by his comment that the child "promptly" has a recur- rence of OME following expulsion of the previous tubes:

10. [7133]   [Attending physician immediately cites prior surgery]
```
 1 Rev:    I don't have any information on him y'know as far as
 2         the frequency of otitis media r' whatever.
 3 Att:    He's a youngster who:: because of recurrent ot- u:h bouts
 4         of otitis media: (.) u::m .h in nineteen eighty seven
 5       → required (.) bilateral myringotomy an- (.) an' post
 6       → (    ) ventilating tubes.
```

```
7          (0.2)
8 Rev:     Mmmm.
9 Att:  →  The tu:bes sh- u::h expe:lled (0.6) someti:me (0.2) middle
10      →  of nineteen ninety, .hh a:nd he promptly had recurrence
11      →  of (0.4) effu:sions despite the use of antibiotic the:rapy,
12         (.) .hh no active infe:ctions but the effusions won't clea:r.
```

In contrast to these cases, other initial mentions of previous surgeries in the patient's history are cited as part of a history of extensive ear problems, though without making an overt connection between the earlier surgeries and the present proposal:

11. [1205]   [Attending physician immediately cites prior surgery]

```
1 Rev:     u:h could you tell me:: u:h (.) something about this y-
2          youngster?=I guess you: wanna put in-=th'-=u:h do a (.)
3          tymp an' tubes on 'im?
4 Att:  →  Okay 'e's had tu:bes uh twi:ce in: u:m (0.4) nineteen
5       →  eighty se:ve:n,=aga:in in u:m (0.2) eighty ni::ne,
6          (0.3) u:h let's see had an ear infection in um (1.0)
7          December and then 'e had 'em aga-=u:h- u:h again:,
8          (.) back in July::, (.) u::hm (0.9) 'e:t's see what
9          else. (0.8) Both u:h (0.4) ears in uh July sho:wed
10         u::m retra:ction with middle ear fluid, '.hh-'
```

In the context of an open-ended request for information about the patient (Boyd 1998), the attending surgeon begins constructing a detailed history of the patient, his relationship with the patient, and his personal, firsthand knowledge of the patient. First, in both instances, is the establishment of prior surgery as part of that rationale. Thus, the attending surgeons display not only that the patients have lengthy and troubled histories of serious ear problems, but that the current situation is not a new one, and so there is *ample precedent for the current decision*. In a majority of these cases (56 per cent) the physician explicitly connected the previous surgeries to the current proposal[6]. Whether explicit or tacit, however, these initial mentions act to legitimate the surgeon's current proposal by displaying a particular historical pattern: each time the patient has had such problems, surgery was the answer; it must, therefore, be the (right) answer now.

While it is evident that a past history of surgery can serve as a starting point from which the attending physician can narrate a history of encounters with the patient, it seems likely that this is at best a secondary motivation for beginning in this way. It is striking that, in cases where the reviewer's initial question does not address previous surgeries, a majority of attending physicians' 'volunteered' mentions of previous surgery occur as the very first statement in the history. This is so despite the history of other potentially describable contacts with the patient both before the initial surgery, and prior to the present conversation. Taken together with the explicit linkage

between previous surgeries and present proposals, the use of these mentions
to anchor a justification for subsequent surgery seems inescapable.

It is clear that these initial comments about prior surgeries can be
persuasive to reviewers. In the following case, the attending physician's
comments induce the reviewer towards a position (arrowed) that sets up a
prospective context for approving the case:

12. [1482]

```
 1 Rev:      I know he's scheduled on the nineteenth
 2 Rev:      fer (.) tu:bes an' u:h .hh he had P E tubes inserted
 3           apparently u:h- eh- were you invo:lved in that I know
 4           you saw him (.) as long ago as July:: of ninety
 5           (0.6)
 6 Rev:      [Did you put his tubes in before?
 7 Att:      [W-
 8 Att:      I'm lookin' here. .hh U::h first of all it's a she::
 9 Rev:      Oh.
10 Att:      An' [u::h she is now about u:h (0.2) nine years old
11 Rev:          [Right.
12 Att:      uh I: uh put her original tubes in .h in December of
13           eighty seven
14 Rev:      Mm hmm. So she's ha:d meh- more than one se:t.
15           (0.2)
16 Att:      The::n lets see how many sets December of eighty seven
17           she had some .hh an' then in Ma:y of eighty ni:ne
18 Rev:      Mm hm.
19 Att:      U::h she had again a bilateral. .h A::nd uh this
20           time her tube is still in her right ear [.hh an'
21 Rev:                                              [Mmhm.
22 Att:      I proposed doin' just her left one.
23 Rev:  →   .hh Is- Is she the ty:pe of patient that just doesn'
24      →    ever clea:r u:p eh even after the tubes come out the
25      →    serous otitis [media just persists¿
26 Att:                   [Ye- Yeah-  yeah-  that's ri:ght she's
27           still got an abnormal tympanogram. .hh An' I- I put
28           in uh- Tee tube...
```

Here the attending physician's account of previous surgeries mobilises the
reviewer towards a generalisation about the patient that defines her as in
need of PE tubes on a long-term basis, and the case was eventually approved
for surgery though it did not satisfy the explicit criteria of the UR firm.

In each of the previous cases, both reviewer and attending surgeon treat
the precedent of prior surgery as (part of) an argument in support of its
subsequent use. This orientation to precedent is particularly marked when
the reviewers, who have no grounds in their mandate for the consideration
of prior surgery, announce their evaluations of the cases. In the context

of both decisions to deny surgery and to recommend it, the reviewing physicians make reference to the notion that prior surgery can justify subsequent surgery – as in (13)–(16).

13. [8401]   Reviewer does not authorise surgery but acknowledges that, for
             the physician, prior surgery is significant]

```
 1 Rev:    U::h (0.4) is there some reason why: you're not
 2         gonna try tuh see if he'll clear up medically? h
 3      →  I realize he's had tubes befo:re, (0.2) but u:h-
 4         (0.1)
 5 Att:    I think that u::h hh you know this has been u:h
 6         duration is u::h about three t' four months hh,
 7         u::m (0.3) I think that u::h hh you know antibiotics
 8         would u:h (0.3) just prolo:ng uh (.) ultimate
 9         tub[e insertion,
10 Rev:       [.H H H H-   Well you might be ri:ght but it- has
11         he been: seen by anyone else u::hr: (0.2) recently
12         be[f- = prior t' this? u:h .h-
13 Att:      [˙˙(He::'s) (          ) I: do:n't kno[:w.
14 Rev:                                            [Yeah.
15 Att:    (                    ) uh, ˙˙ ((too soft to determine
16         whether the noise is the doctor's voice or background
17         noises))
18 Rev:    (0.8) .hh Well the u:h- (.) and you're planning t'
19         do:: uh (.) just PE tubes not (ad'noidectomy) right?
20 Att:    Right.
21 Rev:    Yeah. .hh .hh Well the- u:hm hh (.) most charts
22         don't really:: end up in the physician review area. =
23         Th'- (.) Th' reason this one di:d (.) i:s: u:h an'
24      →  I- I understand where you're comin' from, you're-
25      →  you're- (.) you're thinking since he had tubes
26      →  befo:re that he probably won't clear u:p, .hhh but
27         (.) the question is is there any- is there any
28         reason why the patient would he har:med <i' you
29         tried to treat 'im with antibiotics an' wait u:h >
30         uh little while <t' see if it > does cle:ar since a
31         lot of the effu:sions will? .hh
```

14. [4650]   [Reviewer acknowledges the import of prior surgery]

```
 1 Rev:    we're- we're b- here- we're basically in a
 2         situation where .hh u:m (0.3) if u:h (0.3) i-
 3      →  i- i- if this were the first set uh tubes there
 4         would be no question. I mean the- the- the:- the
 5         panel 'as said that u::h .hh u:h you should wait
 6         at least a couple o' months even if there's a
```

```
7              significant hearing loss after they've had a
8              course of antibiotics uh t' see if it'll clear
9      →      up 'cause most of 'em will. .hh An' th'- In:- In
10     →      this kinda case where they've had them befor:e we
11     →      really don't have it (.) well do:cumented that it-
12     →      that it wouldn't clear up based on prior treatment. =
13             He's only been on the antibiotics for: a fairly
14             short period o' ti:me,
```

In both of these instances, the reviewer addresses the prior surgery as a possible indicator for, or justification of, the current proposal for surgery, even as he is on the way to denying the case. In so doing, the reviewer both acknowledges the legitimacy of the attending surgeon's proposal for surgery, and, by acknowledging it, does his best to mitigate the negative decision. Here, while the acknowledgement of the relevance of prior surgery is a vehicle for mitigating a decision, using it in this way renews the common culture of this medical specialty, and helps to perpetuate the perceived relevance of prior surgery.

This is even more pronounced in cases where the reviewers accepted the precedent as a legitimate override of the criteria. In the next two instances, the reviewers invoked prior surgery as a primary basis for overturning the first-level review and recommending the case for surgery, even though the formal criteria were not satisfied.

15. [1302]   [Reviewer uses prior tubes as basis for overturning decision]

```
1 Rev:    Yeah th- th- th' problem that comes up in a case like this uh
2     →    (.) but uh which, when I heard she had previous tubes I was
3     →    gonna go an' approve it, is that since she's only been on
4          antibiotics for one month we really don't know what'd happen
5          in the next month. Uh when she came back in.
6     →    But with this much hearing loss and previous tubes uh uh eh I'll
7     →    go ahead an' approve it.
```

16. [6190]   [Reviewer uses prior tubes as basis for overturning decision]

```
1 Rev:    Well no I'm not saying what they need or not. I'm just
2     →    saying that uh .hhh I'm gonna go ahead and recommend it
3     →    because uh th fact that u:::h with prior tubes it appeared that he
4     →    did well.
```

In these final instances, prior surgery is explicitly named as the basis for the reviewer's decision to recommend the case for surgery despite the fact that the criteria were not met. Allowed as a sufficient precedent to justify surgery, the myth of prior surgery thoroughly undermines the rational process of the review, while simultaneously being perpetuated through its use.

The summary justifications for approving cases for surgery:
Finally, despite the fact that the UR firm's explicit criteria do not recommend using a history of prior surgery as a basis for their decision making, the reviewing physicians made reference to such surgeries no less than 33 times in their handwritten reports summarising the case for surgery. These entries varied in the extent to which the previous surgeries were explicitly used to justify subsequent surgeries. Thus, in some cases, previous surgeries were simply mentioned as part of a decision-making 'package' of considerations supportive of a decision to approve the case:

17. [Reviewer summary: Case #8658]

    9 year old male w/ eustachian tube insufficiency. Hx of recurrent OM since 1987.
    → Had 5 episodes of SOM until tube insertion late '87. Tubes came out
    → last year and had two episodes AOM in '89 and now has persistent effusion.
    2.5 mos on ABX directed at effusion. Hearing loss 35 db. Discussed cases w/ Dr. L. – approved med. nec.

18. [Reviewer summary: Case #6190]

    → 6 year old child w/last set tubes 6/90 and did well. Seen by Dr. [Name] 5/31/91 w/ SOM and hearing loss. Rx x 1 mo – no improvement on 6/25 visit.
    → In view of recurrent SOM after tubes out, will rec tubes at this time.

Noteworthy in this context is the fact that previous surgeries are mentioned even when the case otherwise merits approval in terms of the UR firm's criteria. For example, Down's Syndrome is an extenuating circumstance mandating surgery. In the following summary, the condition is cited but the previous surgery is also noted:

19. [Reviewer summary: Case #8988]

    7 year old male with Downs syndrome, persistent middle ear effusion, speech problems and hearing loss (20–30db). Effusion now present × 6 weeks.
    → Patient last had tubes in 1986.

Similarly, in (20), the child's prior history of otitic meningitis would be an extenuating circumstance for surgery. Nonetheless, the reviewer adds the references to previous surgeries to bolster the case:

20. [Reviewer summary: Case #1149]

    3 year old child w/ hx otitic meningitis at age 1.
    → Had tubes placed immediately after recovery. Had second set of
    → tubes placed 11/89 which are still in but are now occluded w/ crust.

→ Child did well w/ tubes but now has effusion and had otitis 2 weeks ago.

→ In view of recurring effusion after blockage of tubes and previous severe complication of otitis media, will recommend tubes as medically necessary.

In other cases, however, previous surgeries are explicitly used to justify the present decision favouring surgery, as in (21):

21.   [Reviewer summary: Case #1205]

→ 4 year old child with recurrent episodes of SOM. Previous tubes. Has seen ped and noted to have fluid level again. Child is allergic as well. (   ) Rx for allergy by peds.

→ OK for surgery because of repeated tubes and recurrent fluid.

Through these entries, the reviewers imported the informal ENT culture which they oriented to in their phone calls directly into the official work of the UR firm whose criteria were designed to exclude such considerations from the decision-making process[7]. Prior surgery thus becomes an account for a decision that subverts the very criteria the reviewers were mandated to implement.

As we have suggested, the documentation and discussion of previous surgeries on these patients has a significant impact on the reviewers' decisions. As Table 4 shows there is a strong association between previous surgeries and approvals for current surgeries.

All the inappropriate decisions that were made by the reviewers involved approvals, rather than denials, of cases (Kleinman *et al.* 1997). And, as Table 5 shows, there is a strong association between previous surgeries and decisions to approve new surgeries that are not justified by the UR firm's criteria.

Indeed logistic regression of a range of factors has shown that previous surgeries are the second most significant factor (after patient sex) associated with inappropriate approvals (Kleinman *et al.* 1997: 500, Table 3).

Table 4: *Previous surgeries and outcome of the current review*

Previous surgery	Outcome		
	Deny	*Approve*	*Total*
None	23 (43%)	31 (57%)	54 (100%)
One	7 (21%)	26 (79%)	33 (100%)
More than one	0 (0%)	9 (100%)	9 (100%)
Total	30 (31%)	66 (69%)	96 (100%)

Pearson chi2(2) = 8.8722   Pr = 0.012

Table 5: *Previous surgeries and appropriateness of reviewer decision making*

	Appropriateness of reviewer's decision		
Previous surgery	Appropriate	Inappropriate	Total
None	31 (57%)	23 (43%)	54 (100%)
One	17 (52%)	16 (48%)	33 (100%)
More than one	1 (11%)	8 (89%)	9 (100%)
Total	49 (51%)	47 (49%)	96 (100%)

Pearson chi2(2) = 6.6211   Pr = 0.036

Discussion

This chapter has shown how clinical experience and precedent are treated as legitimate bases for clinical decision making, even in the context of the rationalised process of utilisation review. In this context, where explicit criteria are supposed to be upheld, this use of precedent serves effectively to limit the potential impact of the criteria on clinical practice. As Becker *et al.* noted, experience here is 'used to rule out some of the procedures which have been scientifically established'. Here, the criteria's preference for antibiotic therapy or watchful waiting was frequently ignored in favour of surgery. A history of prior surgery was treated as sufficient to justify current surgery, even though otitis media frequently moderates with age, and evidence to justify the effectiveness of the prior surgery was often scarce. Children with a history of prior tympanostomy surgery were almost 31 times more likely to have their current surgery approved by the reviewers than those with no such history, controlling for a number of important variables (Table 2). In other words 'once a candidate for tympanostomy tubes, always a candidate for tympanostomy tubes'.

Belief in the relevance of prior surgery as grounds for new surgery is widespread in the culture of otolaryngology. As we have documented, communication about previous tympanostomy tube surgeries emerges at every level of the review process and the information that is generated is apt to recur across levels. Thus, in 28 of the 32 (87.5 per cent) cases in which the nurse documented previous surgeries in the scratchpad, there is some further mention or discussion of that in the review conversation. Of the 41 total cases in which references to previous surgeries emerged, the reviewer noted the history of prior surgery in his notes justifying the decision in 33 (80 per cent) of them. The presence of other clinical indications that would represent extenuating circumstances, and which would have been enough to justify approval of the surgery, did not deter the reviewers from noting the prior history of tubes.

There is no evidence in any of our data to suggest that the reviewers or the attending physicians are engaged in any kind of instrumental subversion of the review process. On the contrary, the telephone conversations indicate that the attending physicians sincerely believed that previous surgeries clearly justified future surgery. These beliefs are evidently shared by many of the nurse-reviewers and some of the physician-reviewers as well. The physician-reviewers included prior tympanostomy as part of their 'official' justification to the UR firm, demonstrating a belief in the relevance of this precedent. Thus, the subversion of the UR firm's criteria is subtle and occult. Drawing on a broadly shared, cultural understanding of the role of surgery in treating recurrent illness, and found at all levels of the review process, prior surgery is treated by all parties as a critical and consequential finding that is relevant to the decision at hand. Its relevance is treated by all parties as immediate, and its status as an account is treated as unproblematic. In many ways, this is a circular self-validating belief functioning at a near-presuppositional level in many of these review conversations (Pollner 1987). It is unproblematically used to justify approving cases for surgery, and special pleading is involved in defeating its relevance for surgery.

From the perspective of the reviewers, who are peers of the reviewed physicians and stand in a potentially collegial relationship to them, rejection of the relevance of prior surgery is difficult to manage and is only attempted when the reviewers tried to justify denying the case for surgery. Not only is the relevance of prior surgery for future decisions shared within the ENT culture, reference to it by the reviewers is a means both of building a collegial relationship with the attending physicians, and positioning themselves as sympathetic to the attending physicians' proposals for the case (Boyd 1998). Moreover, denials of these cases were often conflictual and emotionally stressful for the reviewers (Boyd 1997). The history of prior surgery provided a consensually validated rationale for approving the case in the context of the review process, even in the case of discord with the criteria. Thus the invocation of prior surgery both exerted pressure on the reviewers to approve the case, while making it easier for them to do so.

Conclusion

This is a study of the ways in which the informal culture of medical practice, with its essentially autonomous and particularistic ways of making medical decisions, is introduced into a system of utilisation review that was designed to embody the highest standards of scientific rationality. Through the interactional administration of utilisation review, this informal culture leaks into the putatively technocratic system of evidence-based medicine, inserting into both the process and its outcomes a kind of collegial mythology that, from the point of view of scientific medicine, is based on half-truths or no truth at all.

Although this is an examination of some of the practices by which physicians perpetuate a particular medical myth, this study also reveals the complexities, as well as some of the difficulties, involved in efforts to ration health care. Hunter (1997) and Mechanic (1995), among others, have suggested that forms of explicit rationing, such as the utilisation review process examined here, are especially vulnerable to duplicity or efforts to "game the system" as physicians (and other professionals) attempt to circumvent explicit criteria. While that may be the case, this study shows that the implementation of explicit criteria may be highly vulnerable to more subtle means of subversion based on shared and quasi-presuppositional beliefs within the medical profession. As long as these beliefs remain entrenched within the culture of medicine, the implementation of efforts to ration and rationalise health care will remain susceptible to such occult subversion.

This chapter has provided evidence of the subversion of scientifically and bureaucratically rational decision making by the members of a medical specialty. However, these data were gathered at the beginning of the UR firm's development of prospective utilisation review. The reviewers were often faced with attending physicians who were deeply unhappy with the very idea of utilisation review, and especially its prospective use. As one otolaryngologist lamented, 'I really appreciate medicine being played by someone three thousand miles away from the patient, [who has] never seen the patient and then decides what is good for the patient'. Others, whose proposals for surgery were denied, lambasted the review process: 'What you're doing actually has nothing to do with medical care. It has absolutely nothing to do with quality of care. It has to do with saving a buck'. It is in this context, of course, that the reviewers came to overturn about two-thirds of the first-level reviews and approved the cases for surgery, most of them inappropriately.

The relative inefficiency of the review process as a means of rationing care was quite visible to the UR firm. Nonetheless, it can be suggested that such an inefficient and dysfunctional review process has long-term value from the perspective of those who would ration care. These data represent the introduction to attending physicians of a process to hold their medical decisions accountable in terms of explicit criteria. While both the attending physicians and the reviewing physicians collaborated in subverting these criteria, it is possible that another, and deeper, process of occult subversion was at work. The object of this subversion is the very notion of physician autonomy in medical decision making, and the incipient replacement of the collegial regulation of medical practice with that of a bureaucratic process. Indeed the rationing of health care in the name of quality of health care must ultimately depend on co-opting medical professionals to relinquish their autonomy. The use of physician-reviewers, who share mythical and cultural beliefs with the attending physician, to initiate this process may actually have been effective in contributing to this co-option. In this way, the dysfunctional aspects of the review process described here may have made a contribution to the changing pattern of practices in medical decision making in managed care.

Acknowledgments

We are grateful to Value Health Sciences for unrestricted access to the data, and to Drs. Jacqueline Kosecoff, Robert W. Dubois, and Debra Kile at VHS and to Dr. Helen Blumen, formerly of VHS. Dr. Ed Park of RAND provided invaluable assistance in creating the original study design and the sampling scheme. Dr. Robert H. Brook provided important conceptual and practical insights.

Notes

1   At the time of the decision, the surgeons were given an 800-number to call to initiate appeal proceedings. The physician-reviewer was not involved in the appeal decision.

2   Potential complications of tubes include perforation of the tympanic membrane, scarring and permanent low-grade hearing loss [Kleinman 1997], as well as the general threat from anesthesia.

3   A study by Kleinman *et al.* (1994) of some 4000 tympanostomy surgeries found that 41 per cent were appropriate, 36 per cent were equivocal and 23 per cent were inappropriate in terms of criteria described below.

4   The Agency for Healthcare Research and Quality (AHRQ, formerly the Agency for Healthcare Policy and Research, AHCPR) has also issued national guidelines for the appropriate use of tympanostomy tubes for the management of otitis media. Kleinman (1997) demonstrates that the AHCPR guidelines are much more restrictive than the UR firm's criteria, both in general and when applied to this population.

5   The official extenuating circumstance involves cleft palate, not lip. This issue later became the focus of discussion in the review.

6   In a total of seven out of 16 cases in which attending physicians initiated mentions of prior tubes they associated previous surgeries with positive effects (the patient 'did well'), or associated current difficulties with loss of benefits from previous tubes which had 'become extruded' or 'blocked'. Such associations were more common when attending-initiated mentions of previous surgeries occurred at the beginning of the review process, rather than as a more 'en passant' or embedded mention as part of the child's medical history. Assertions of medical benefits associated with prior surgeries occurred in less than 10 per cent of the cases in which reviewers questioned attending physicians about prior surgeries.

7   The reactions to these non-legitimate reviewer justifications on the part of the UR firm and the third party payers it represents are not known. The UR firm had records of each reviewer's approval rates and may, on occasion, have examined individual reviewer records. However the volume of reviews likely precluded detailed analysis of reviewer justifications.

References

Becker, H., Geer, B., Hughes, E. and Strauss, A. (1961) *Boys in White: Student Culture in Medical School*. New Brunswick, NJ: Transaction Publishers.

Berg, M. (1997) *Rationalizing Medical Work: Decision-Support Techniques and Medical Practices*. Cambridge, Mass: The MIT Press.

Bluestone, C.D. and Klein, J.O. (1988) *Otitis Media in Infants and Children*. Philadelphia, PA: WB Saunders Co.

Boyd, E. (1997) *Constructing Histories and Negotiating Care: Professional Discourse during Medical Peer Review*. Unpublished PhD dissertation, University of California, Los Angeles.

Boyd, E. (1998) Bureaucratic authority in the 'company of equals': the interactional management of medical peer review, *American Sociological Review*, 63, 200–24.

Brook, R.H., Chassin, M.R., Fink, A., Solomon, D.H., Kosecoff, J. and Park, R.E. (1986) A method for the detailed assessment of the appropriateness of medical technologies, *International Journal of Technology Assessment in Health Care*, 2, 53–63.

Cantekin, E., McGuire, T. and Griffith, T. (1991) Antimicrobial therapy for otitis media with effusion ('secretory' otitis media), *Journal of the American Medical Association*, 266, 3309–17.

Hunter, D.J. (1997) *Desperately Seeking Solutions: Rationing Health Care*. London: Longman.

Kleinman, L. (1997) Off the (bench)mark? The clinical characteristics of insured American children proposed to receive tympanostomy tubes, 1990–91, compared to the recommendations of the 1994 AHCPR Guideline for Otitis Media with Effusion. Paper presented at Pediatric Academic Societies National Meeting, May 1997.

Kleinman, L., Kosecoff, J., Dubois, R. and Brook, R. (1994) The medical appropriateness of tympanostomy tubes proposed for children younger than 16 years in the United States, *Journal of the American Medical Association* 271, 16, 1250–5.

Kleinman, L., Boyd, E. and Heritage, J. (1997) Adherence to prescribed explicit criteria during utilization review: an analysis of the communications between attending and reviewing physicians, *Journal of the American Medical Association*, 278, 6, 497–501.

Mechanic, D. (1995) Dilemmas in rationing health care services: the case for implicit rationing, *British Medical Journal*, 310, 1655–9.

Pollner, M. (1987) *Mundane Reason: Reality in Everyday and Sociological Discourse*. Cambridge: Cambridge University Press.

9

Clinical actions and financial constraints: the limits to rationing intensive care

Irvine Lapsley and Kath Melia

Introduction

The provision of health care in the UK can be characterised as a situation of excess demand. Regardless of the amount of resources devoted to health care, there is never enough capacity to service demands, as evidenced, for example, by lengthening waiting lists. In the face of excess demands, one management response is to ration activities. Such rationing may be shaped by historical antecedents, the configuration, for instance, of units within hospitals (the space and beds available to them) and of hospitals themselves. Other ways in which rationing is shaped include new management priorities, a change in patterns of clinical care; and, most notably, a shortage of resources to finance increases in, or changing patterns of, care.

In this chapter we examine the provision of intensive care in the context of excess demand and explore the limits to the managerial option of rationing intensive care. There are a number of limits to the explicit introduction of rationing of intensive care. This is a branch of medicine in which clinicians are confronted with life or death decisions; it is a relatively young discipline and one which lacks robust, sophisticated planning tools, which would facilitate the rationing of activities by aligning finance available with the quantification of clinical priorities. The nature of intensive care is such that it fosters strong clinical groupings which provide a basis for the resistance of attempts to ration intensive care.

In this chapter we contend that the debate on rationing is often expressed in terms of its presence or absence (see *e.g.* Rothman 1992). This particular perspective does not give due weight to the actions of clinicians in redefining the boundaries which are imposed in an attempt to ration their activities. We distinguish between two types of rationing of health care: *hard rationing* and *soft rationing*. By *hard rationing* we mean a situation in which the scope and scale of activities are limited by binding constraints which may be financial or physical (for example, numbers of beds, availability of staff, budgets). *Soft rationing*, on the other hand, is a situation in which there may exist general constraints (of a financial or physical nature) which limit activities, but which may be attenuated by the actions of clinical managers. In *hard rationing*, absolute limits may be observed which limit the range and scope of activities: in *soft rationing*, the actions of clinical managers and their ingenuity in redrawing or shifting apparently binding constraints determine whether a situation of *hard capital rationing* will take hold. The evidence of this chapter suggests that the nature of intensive care is such that *soft rationing* is most likely to work for this field of health care.

Method of investigation

We examine the phenomenon of *soft rationing* in intensive care by the use of both primary and secondary sources, this examination is conducted along three dimensions. We use secondary sources for an a priori examination of both the nature of intensive care and the attempts at calculation and modelling of intensive care. These are important factors in understanding the limits to rationing in intensive care. We seek first, to determine whether there are prima facie intrinsic aspects of intensive care which make the imposition of absolute limits on resources and activities (*hard rationing*) unlikely. Secondly, we explore calculation and modelling of intensive care because the ability to model activities with precision is an important aspect of the development of sophisticated budgeting systems which would present the possibility for a more explicit consideration of the financial constraint in a situation of *hard rationing*, for example, activity based management (Antos 1992).

These two aspects of intensive care are necessary, but not sufficient, grounds for a situation of *hard rationing* to develop. A crucial third element can be found in the dynamics of complex organisations such as the intensive care unit (ICU) namely, the motivation and behaviour of key actors in these settings. This third dimension of *soft rationing*, the actions of clinicians, is examined using our primary source data from our study of three ICUs. A multiple case study design (Yin 1994) enables us to gain an understanding of clinical actions in the face of possible rationing. The development of informal networks within and between these hospital units represents an important element of clinical behaviour. We examine this aspect of the behaviour of clinicians which has been described in the literature in terms of informal networks, focusing on the work of Granovetter (1973, 1982, 1985, 1992) to explore the functioning of these networks in intensive care.

Table 1 shows background data on the intensive care units (ICUs) included in this part of the study.

Interviews were undertaken with clinicians, that is, consultant anaesthetists in charge of the ICUs; nursing service managers; experienced ICU nurses working on the units in senior clinical nursing posts and as direct

Table 1: *Background data of case study sites*[1]

1. *McIntyre Teaching*	2. *Campbell General*	3. *McDonald General*
• 10 bedded unit (to increase to 12)	• 4 bedded unit	• 6 bedded unit
• part of Anaesthetics and Operating Theatres directorate	• part of Surgical directorate	• part of Surgical directorate
• £2M budget	• £800K budget	• £1.5M budget
• 8 consultants	• 5 consultants	• 5 consultants
• 70 intensive care nurses	• 28 intensive care nurses	• 42 intensive care nurses

[1] extracts from the data are numbered 1, 2, 3 as in this table.

carers; management accountants; and hospital finance managers. These interviews were conducted as in-depth qualitative, open-ended exchanges on a specified set of topics to maximise our understanding of the interplay between finance, accounting and the clinical perspective (Blumer 1969, Glaser and Strauss 1967, Hughes 1971, Denzin 1989). Each of these interviews lasted for around one hour and 30 minutes. In total, there were interviews with 21 people at the three study sites. These interviews were assisted by the use of real life constructs (Lapsley and Llewellyn, 1995) which are assemblages of information from actual organisational practices in intensive care which are situationally specific.

Our data comprise a series of interview transcripts and various accounting data, spreadsheets and reports to which we were given access. These data were supplemented by an examination of the accounting details, budget profiles, staffing levels and other documentation and policies, adding a quantitative aspect to the study. We also examined reports and statistics concerning the costs of provision of intensive care and an analysis of the clinical outcomes of the service. The national figures on which these reports are based provided a context within which to understand the management of cost in the ICUs studied. Our analysis has taken the form of scrutiny of the transcripts and pursuing the main themes which emerged.

The limits to rationing: the nature of intensive care

Since the establishment of intensive care services in the 1960s, there has been significant growth in intensive care facilities. This phenomenon is a reflection of changes in clinical practice: clinicians undertaking medical interventions expect to have an intensive care facility available to patients in need, as a necessary part of modern care (Edbrooke *et al.* 1999). The rate of growth of expenditure in this area is often greater than that of the health care system, as a whole (Birnbaum, 1986; Singer *et al.* 1983; Edbrooke *et al.*

1999). The increase in resources devoted to intensive care is, in part, because of the relatively high operating costs of intensive care units (Spivack 1987).

Zussman (1992) in a study of medical ethics in intensive care units notes that medicine is more constrained by the law than was once the case. This is symptomatic of the sensitivity of the ICU case load, where clinicians are often presented with complex cases without predictable outcomes. Similarly, nurses working in intensive care are concerned with ethical issues, and these too become extant in the daily working practices of the intensive care unit (Chambliss 1996, Melia 2001). These sociological analyses of the daily experience of ethical issues in the ICU underline the fact that clinical decisions need to be justified on moral grounds.

There are major ethical challenges for clinicians at the micro level of the ICU as they deal with specific patients. Swenson (1992) expresses the kinds of dilemmas with which they are confronted:

> Most ethical problems that arise in the care of ICU patients have to do with the provision or discontinuation of particular therapies. Should life-sustaining mechanical ventilation be discontinued for this comatose woman? Should dialysis be initiated for this man with an inoperable brain tumour? The decision to withhold or withdraw treatment is usually based on a consensus amongst patients, families, and physicians (1992: 551).

Swenson's description captures the nature of the decisions to be made, their complexity is often due to the multiple pathology in ICU cases. He also conveys the difficult process of making such decisions when several 'voices' are present. All of this makes the ICU an unsuitable case for the imposition of arbitrary activity levels, in other words an unsuitable case for *hard rationing*.

Resource availability, however, impinges on the clinical management of ICUs. For example, the physical configuration of available ICU beds, and related skilled nursing staffing capacity are important constraints on the effectiveness of ICUs. Swenson expands upon the manner in which this can impact upon clinical practice in ICUs:

> ... there are situations in which resource scarcity becomes the central issue. If there are too few ICU beds to accommodate all who need them, how should they be distributed? Is it ever permissible to withdraw needed ICU care from one patient to make room for another? (1992: 551).

These circumstances point to possible ethical dilemmas for clinical managers of ICUs. The sensitivity of the cases considered, however, makes ICUs unlikely candidates for *hard rationing*. The clinical management of specific cases and of specific facilities in the manner described by Swenson fits our definition of *soft rationing*: to which we return in the following section.

The limits to rationing: calculation and clinical practice

The aforementioned problems for budgeting for intensive care – its unpredictable nature, the increasing demand – are accentuated by the unavailability of robust systems of measuring the severity of the cases which ICU teams handle. In any attempt at rationing, a major difficulty with intensive care is the problem of measuring activity and outputs. A priori, the devising of scoring systems which capture key dimensions of the activities of ICUs would facilitate the process of rationing care insofar as this would provide information on needs which could be matched to available resources. The development of robust information on activities would provide a basis for the construction of workload-based budgets with the twin implications of greater precision in budget-setting for ICUs and the possibility, if desired, of tightening the financial constraint within which these units operate. This would contrast with current practice in budget-setting which is essentially based on historical patterns of expenditure and is, at best, incremental (Lapsley 1994).

There has been considerable effort by researchers in health care to devise scoring systems which would assist clinical managers of intensive care units. However, as shown below, neither of the main scoring systems (or their variants) is sufficiently robust to enable detailed planning which would facilitate aligning activity levels with financial allocations and, thereby, raising the possibility for *hard rationing* to develop. The first was the Therapeutic Intervention Scoring System (TISS), devised by Cullen *et al.* (1974) as a management tool to cost the processes of care. It was designed to measure clinical workload. A second is the Acute Physiology and Chronic Health Evaluation (APACHE) originally devised by Knaus *et al.* (1981) to measure severity of illness.

Therapeutic Intervention Scoring System (TISS)
TISS has been used to determine nursing workloads and to investigate the costs of intensive care (Jacobs 1996). This might be thought to be especially relevant, as a major part of the ICU budget is taken up by nursing salaries. However, there are problems of internal consistency in using a single score which is made up of a complex of components. At the individual patient level, TISS cannot be used as a predictive tool because the individual circumstances of each case vary too widely. It may be used by management as a tool for costing the processes of care and to assist in making resource allocation decisions (Miranda *et al.* 1998), but it is a rough and ready rather than a precise tool.

Acute Physiology and Chronic Health Evaluation (APACHE)
Knaus *et al.* (1981), working on the idea that an indication of the variation from the norm on several key physiological measures would provide an assessment of the severity of the illness, devised the APACHE severity of

disease scoring system. APACHE II and a further modification, APACHE III, are tools designed to enable evaluation of performance of ICUs and of new and existing therapies.

APACHE is not an individual case specific predictor. APACHE gives an indication of the successes of intensive care and allows comparison of results and mortality rates between different ICUs. But as a tool it cannot be used for decisions concerning individual patients and so is of no day-to-day use to intensive care clinicians in the management of their service, nor to accountants in the management of budgets. So whilst, theoretically, the dynamic use of APACHE II should allow predictions for survival and give grounds for withdrawal of treatment, and so effect savings in terms of human suffering and resources, the shortcomings of the method and the fact that we are dealing with human life has to lead to the conclusion that these scoring systems cannot be used as a basis for such decisions.

Atkinson et al. (1994) used modified APACHE II organ failure scores to make predictions of the outcomes of 3,600 patients. Of the 137 patients predicted to die, 131 (95.6 per cent) did so within 90 days of discharge:

Patients predicted to die stayed 1,492 days in intensive care and incurred 16.7 per cent of the total intensive care expenditure.

Their conclusions point up the difficulty of translating these scoring systems into managerial or clinical decisions. According to Atkinson and his colleagues:

If used prospectively, this algorithm has the potential to indicate the futility of continued intensive care but at the cost of one in 20 patients who would survive if the intensive care were continued. (Atkinson et al. 1994: 1203)

This verdict demonstrates clearly the ethical limitations to the utility of this model.

Although on the face of it these scoring systems appear to provide very precise measures of patients' morbidity, they are of no use to clinicians with respect to managing individual cases. One problem for the management of the ICU budget is that accounting is about quantification. There are no sophisticated workload models readily available to assist in this and the only means of clinical quantification that exist to date are the scoring systems (TISS and APACHE), neither of which is sufficiently precise or refined for use in budget construction. As a consequence, the professional judgement of the clinicians provides a 'precision' which available budgetary numbers cannot, and so their views prevail.

The very complexity of intensive care, as an activity, means that the costing information available within ICUs is not very sophisticated (Miranda et al. 1998). The most obvious means by which accounting information could come to bear on the activities of intensive care units would be as a crude budgetary constraint in the form of *hard rationing*. In this respect, it is the response of clinicians to the formal language of new style hospital management, namely budgets, costs and cash constraints (Lapsley 1994), that is a crucial determinant of what rationing means in practice.

The limits to rationing: clinical actions

The third element to the limits of rationing in intensive care is that of the actions of the clinicians in the discharge of their duties. Our data show a willingness on the part of clinicians to engage with each other and with the management of their hospitals and beyond to relax constraints, physical or budgetary, which if left in place would have been an acceptance of *hard rationing*. We examine examples of this networking behaviour in the face of limited resources, below, but first we examine the financial situation of the ICUs in our study.

The intensive care units at all three of the Scottish hospitals included in this part of this study are in financial difficulties. Every unit has higher expenditure than the amount of monies allocated to them as part of the annual budgetary cycle. At McIntyre, the intensive care unit had an overspend of 15 per cent of the budget; at Campbell, the intensive care unit had an overspend of six per cent and at McDonald, the overspend was 13 per cent. In part, this situation is a function of the budget-setting process, which, as noted above, tends to be historical in the NHS. It is also a function of the uncertainty associated with predicting activity levels in an emergency-driven service. Increasing expectations of, and demands for, intensive care places stresses on the resources allocated to these units, and this adds to the problems. A possible consequence of this imprecise process is that crude budgetary limits could contain or curtail the activities of these intensive care units: a case of *hard rationing*. This crude form of rationing, however, does not occur in the intensive care service because it would appear that there is no simple acceptance of historical levels of resources on the part of the health care professionals who work together in their commitment to intensive care.

The ways in which clinicians have responded to constraints on available resources has been to act in concert in ways which foster their goals in clinical practice. They work together in a network which has both formal and informal elements, where team commitment and support and professional understanding produce the solidarity of a network. The use of networks has been advocated as a general frame of reference for the exploration of the interface between the world of health care professionals and that of management (Ferlie and Pettigrew 1996). The concept of social networks (Granovetter 1973, 1982, 1985, 1992) has informed our study. Granovetter (1992) argues that organisations may be shaped in quite different ways, depending on the configuration of the interpersonal networks of leading actors. In Granovetter's terms, attempts at purposive action are embedded in concrete, ongoing systems of social relations. In the intensive care provision that we studied we found tangible evidence for the existence of social networks in the interactions between clinical teams and the management of the hospitals in which they are located. Of particular interest to our exploration of networks was the construction of a benchmarking report for all three ICUs; this entailed a specific dialogue with management and the funding authorities. These kinds of activities reveal strong agency pressures within the professional grouping to relax financial and resource constraints and, thereby, to induce *soft rationing* situations.

Clinical networks in action: (1) the clinician – management interface
The ICUs included in this study, when confronted with shortages of resources or financial constraints, displayed the characteristics of Granovetter's subgroups. One notable characteristic of the ICU clinicians' activity was the manner in which the clinical staff had engaged with finance staff on the question of the legitimacy of financial constraints. This joint action, which is evidence of the strength and shared values of the social network, resulted in the removal of apparently binding constraints and a shift from a potential situation of *hard rationing* to one of *soft rationing*. This resistance to apparently binding financial constraints manifests itself in a number of ways: the discourse with finance professionals and persuading them of the clinical perspective; the taking of key decisions on care with significant financial implications; and the active management of the physical constraint of the numbers of beds (with appropriate staff) available for intensive care.

The following data extract demonstrates the approach of the network in action. When asked by the researchers 'does it ever come to the point where you really do have to say, "well, look we really can't do this", that this would cause you worry?' the consultant anaesthetist at Campbell General said:

> The answer to that is no. If it is in the patient's interests and we can argue our case cogently that there are no other alternatives then that goes ahead. It has to *[Anaesthetist 2]*.

The accountants with specific responsibilities for the financial management of ICUs who were interviewed in this study had become part of the social network and were sympathetic to this clinical view. These accountants were also sensitive to the deficiencies of historically-constructed budgets, particularly in intensive care. At McIntyre Teaching Hospital, the accountant with responsibility for the budget construction for intensive care described the budget setting, as follows:

> It largely rolls forward from year to year. How it was derived originally is probably lost in the passing of time, but it's usually done by activity *[Management accountant 1]*.

and in response to a query about attempts to vary this, he responded:

No, we don't build up from the bottom. There's no bottom up budget.
It's primarily rolled forward and adjusted for significant variances.
Don't mention zero based budgeting. It was mentioned a few years ago.
I'm all for zero based budgeting, but give me a break [*Management
accountant 1*].

This response may seem somewhat negative, but it is not exceptional. When
the management accountant at Campbell General Hospital was appointed,
he built up a zero based budget – a needs-driven statement of the resources
requested for adequate funding of the intensive care unit. This accountant
described the impact of this initiative:

... Effectively we had a zero based budget and we did this some two
years ago, where we effectively built the budget for the whole directorate
from scratch. We started with a white (sic) sheet of paper. And we built
the budget from scratch. Needless to say, when we did that, it blew up
some fairly significant differences.... The trouble was, we didn't
actually get the funding, that reflected needs. So, I said to them: Guys,
this is where we believe we need to be, and here are the figures, however,
we don't believe we're going to get all of this because of efficiency savings,
funding ceilings, new formulae for resource allocation [*Management
accountant 2*].

According to this accountant, his clinical colleagues' response was to say:

Oh what's the point of doing all this. We may as well just run as we
always run, and hell mend them, we'll never get the resources we need to
run the show and that's the end of it [*Management accountant 2*].

It is interesting to note that the accountant at the third hospital, McDonald
General, was in the process of trying to shift its practices from historically-
based to zero-based budgets. In his scheme, budgets were being constructed
based on outturns[1] to get a more accurate understanding of the cost base for
the hospital. When questioned, however, he conceded that the overspend
at McDonald General's intensive care unit would be part of its budget
for next year – with the exception of non-recurring items (which would
be slight, given the structure of intensive care costs, which are dominated
by staff costs). This tells us about the discourse between accountants and
clinicians and the resultant relaxation of a seemingly binding budgetary
constraint.

   The description above paints a picture of accountants recognising, readily,
the limitations of the financial constraints which are imposed on intensive
care. Furthermore, as the exchange with the accountant at Campbell Hospital

cited above shows, the clinical members of intensive care teams are not passive in their acceptance of financial constraints.

Within ICU teams there are several possible responses to the threat of financial constraints. First, there is scope for engagement with the finance staff on appropriate levels of funding by the consultant with administrative responsibilities in the ICU and by other consultant colleagues. This did occur, and the clinicians were all articulate advocates of the case for additional resources for intensive care. However, further scope for action lies in the straightforward taking of a clinical decision, on clinical grounds. We have instances of these clinicians taking decisions which were costly, and allowing the needs of the patient to override financial considerations. One example given was a patient with extensive injury, who was treated with an extremely expensive product chosen on grounds of clinical effectiveness. This was an expensive treatment choice and the ICU was already over budget. The consultant in charge, however, with the agreement of the clinical director, decided to go ahead with this treatment. The accountant was unaware of this until the outturn figures on the unit's financial statements registered the significant overspend. The patient with the extensive injury provides a good example of how the clinical staff can act to relax apparent budget constraints. This was an example of resisting *hard rationing*.

In terms of physical constraints, the most obvious one was that of staffed ICU beds. Each of these intensive care units included in this study had a fixed number of beds with an appropriate level of staffing for an intensive care unit. The clinical teams managed this constraint by the active monitoring of patients' progress. This might mean the discharge of a patient from the ICU:

> The other point I would make, on a personal level, we were brought up in a climate that doesn't play bed games. Basically if we can stagger you out of ITU, you're staggered out of ITU, which I don't think is prevalent in a lot of hospitals *[Consultant anaesthetist-in-charge 1]*.

It may also mean the relaxation of the physical constraint of bed space by the temporary extension of intensive care into high dependency units or recovery areas, which we found in our study, as the following comment from one of the clinicians illustrates:

> One of the uncertainties is that we don't know if there is a bed available for the patient when we set off.... This stresses our staff – medical and nursing. It might have to be a bed for the patient in the High Dependency Unit. At the end of the day we sort it out *[Consultant anaesthetist-in-charge 1]*.

The same clinician went on to expand upon how ICU teams work with colleagues in related areas to relax the binding constraint of bed numbers:

If you look in the HDU [High Dependency Unit] a lot of people are in hospital who are teetering along hoping they will be all right, and likewise discharging people from ITU in that way. We don't have good information on that, we are starting to collect that a bit more formally, which we haven't done in the past *[Consultant anaesthetist-in-charge 1]*.

This pattern of making optimal use of available facilities is based upon these sub-groups or sub-networks in ICU monitoring bed usage and acting decisively to maximise usage. This pattern is repeated in all of the intensive care units within the three hospitals included in this study. There is yet a further element of evidence which demonstrates that these clinical networks are in action as active forces for the relaxation of *hard* constraints thus rendering them *soft*. In addition to the intra-hospital bed management activities described above, there are inter-hospital arrangements between the ICUs sited in the three hospitals. So, where a given hospital is unable to overcome the constraint of its bed capacity by discharge or transfer to a high dependency unit, it may call upon clinical colleagues at these other hospitals, as part of this clinical network, to enlist their assistance in coping with these patients who would otherwise not receive intensive care.

These practices involve the intensive care staff taking calculated risks as their main strategy for ensuring that, even though intensive care resources are limited, they are available to those patients in need. These clinical actions are taken in situations of physical constraints, yet the resource limitation does not impinge directly on the clinicians, who follow through their clinical decisions by collaboration and teamwork with clinicians in related areas (high dependency, the recovery area) and seek to relax the physical constraint of bed availability which could otherwise ration intensive care.

A strong team ethos, consistent with network behaviour, is exhibited by these intensive care teams (in Granovetter's terms, a strong sub-network) in their multidisciplinary approach to care. Where democratic, consensual parts of the organisation (such as these intensive care teams) exist, there are tenacious, strong sub-groups (Granovetter 1982). It has long been recognised that the complexity of hospitals as organisations may lead to the creation of stable sub-networks or sub groups (Granovetter 1985). This description is apt for the ICU teams at all three of the hospitals we studied, as they are characterised by close interpersonal relationships and a strong team effort. This team effort showed through in the shared commitment of the different professionals – nurses, doctors, accountants and managers – involved in intensive care. These networks operated in such a way that they reinforced the resistance to the possibility of *hard rationing* by focusing on the relaxation of physical and financial constraints.

Clinical networks in action: (2) the benchmarking exercise
A second response to constraints on their activities was for the health care professionals across the three ICUs in this study to draw upon their own

resources as a network in order to challenge and engage with the management of hospitals. Within the clinical intensive care team there were members of staff with MBA qualifications (one at McIntyre Teaching, one at Campbell General). These members of staff display a detailed knowledge of the budgetary process, which enabled them to engage with management. It was these management-literate clinical members of staff who were instrumental in taking these informal networks a stage further by being involved in a benchmarking exercise, which investigated bed usage, staffing levels, and budgetary allocations in the ICUs across all three hospitals.

Benchmarking is a management tool and reflects both current management thought (Cox and Thompson 1998) and the practices of oversight bodies[2] in the public sector (Accounts Commission 1999). This benchmarking exercise provides a very clear and important example of the intensive care team working as a social network. At the inter-hospital level, however, the social network of intensive care professionals exists mainly at the clinical level. This dimension of the network is based on weaker ties than are found in the intra-hospital, multi-disciplinary team. At the inter-hospital level, these clinicians know each other, but meet infrequently. One setting in which these clinicians meet is their local intensive care society, which meets relatively infrequently. However, it does produce an annual report to which all intensive care units contribute. Also, these clinicians all belong to the same social background, read the same professional journals and have in common the membership of a powerful professional group. Nevertheless, these intermittent contacts and weak ties may actually strengthen the operation of the network when it is necessary to call upon it (Granovetter 1973). In our study we found evidence to suggest that a strong network, based on weak ties, was operating when the clinicians from the three ICUs collaborated on the benchmarking exercise.

The behaviour of the clinicians within the three ICUs in this study bears the hallmarks of a social network (Granovetter 1973), that is to say, the clinicians exhibited trust and recognised that they were dependent upon one another. This clinical network was based on 'weak ties' and exercised professional autonomy in the pursuit of additional resources to reduce the likelihood of having to ration intensive care services.

Alter (1990) has argued that the influence of conflict on networking can be important for cohesion within networks. In this regard, the continuation of *soft rationing* in the face of persistent excess demand can build up pressures and create conflict with the overall system or bureaucracy. Conflict can be seen as a necessary condition for the collaborative success of the health care professionals in the network. The benchmarking report had been produced in order to compare resources for the ICUs in the hospitals providing intensive care in the Region. We first heard reference made to this in an interview with one of the managers:

we are using it [quantitative data] at the moment because we're reviewing ITU services across the Region, so this kind of information is the stuff we are looking for in terms of resource allocation. Now, not in terms of 'we have this number of patients who are this sick, therefore we need this money', because that is a wee bit too simple. But by comparing ourselves, for example using APACHE II scores, we have been able to demonstrate that the patients who arrive in our ITU, although it's a smaller ITU than at McDonald General and McIntyre Teaching, so we can use the information to that level, although the number of patients is quite different, but they are as sick coming here. So using it for that is therefore arguing that if there is any resource to be divvied up you know, a proportion must come this way *[Manager 2]*.

As we noted above, benchmarking is currently a fashionable management tool which originated in the private sector, but which is being used increasingly in the public services (Accounts Commission 1999). However, the way in which the management-literate clinicians used benchmarking is of particular interest. In the face of increasing numbers of patients and a continuous striving to manage or relax existing constraints, which would have effectively rationed the intensive care provided by these clinical teams, there was a desire in these ICUs to make a bid for a significant increase in the level of resources. However, instead of producing a management-driven report which examined the costs of provision, these intensive care teams produced a report which emphasised clinical considerations. The clinicians' reports emphasised the severity of illness of patients, patient flows – admissions, discharges, bed occupancy – and staffing levels. Unlike a benchmarking exercise as an accountant would understand it, in this report operating costs were given lower prominence and appeared as an addendum to the report.

The very act of compiling the data and comparing the profiles of these three ICUs required a significant amount of time and effort on the part of these clinical teams. But the compilation of the report was only the beginning. Ultimately, their report brought additional resources to these ICUs which permitted additional fully-funded (staffed) beds for intensive care. However, the clinicians acting in concert as a network had to take this report to the management in each hospital for additional resources, only to be informed that no additional resources were available. These clinicians then took their report to Health Board level. Again, they were denied additional resources. Ultimately, the report was taken to the central government department responsible for health care, where it was agreed that additional resources be allocated.

These characteristics of the behaviour of ICU consultants conform to the patterns expected of network-like behaviour. There is clear interdependence between the constituents of this network (Hakansson and Johanson 1993). The professional relationships have persisted and exhibited some degree of longevity (Powell 1991). Also there is clear evidence of mutual adaptation and complementarity in the behaviour of these ICU teams (Johanson and

Mattson 1991; Hakansson and Johanson 1993). The willingness of intensive care teams to seek to redefine apparent binding constraints (*hard rationing*) in order to soften their effect reaffirms our characterisation of these clinical teams as resilient. Our findings confirm Granovetter's theses that weak ties can lead to very strong network characteristics and behaviour. This is further confirmed by the final outcome of this protracted engagement for resources: the major beneficiary of this struggle was the ICU at Campbell General Hospital. The most prestigious hospital (McIntyre) also had strong claims for additional resources. However, this outcome was accepted by all of the parties concerned, without dispute: a 'victory' for the network in action.

Conclusion

This study has reported on the impact of social networks on rationing in intensive care. We have distinguished between two types of rationing: *hard rationing*, in which activities face absolute limits, whether these are physical or financial constraints; and *soft rationing*, in which apparently tight physical or financial constraints can be relaxed by the actions of key actors within the organisation. We characterise the situation confronting the intensive care units in this study as one of *soft rationing*.

There are important facets of the work of intensive care which are preconditions for social networks to be able to exercise the kind of influence which can lift constraints and move ICUs from *hard* to *soft rationing*. One significant element of this is the very nature of intensive care itself, which entails dealing with complex cases involving multiple pathology, where the prediction of outcomes for patients is extremely difficult. The nature of intensive care means that there are ethical considerations associated with the decisions to treat or to withdraw intensive care from patients. These ethical issues impact on the daily lives of all clinical staff in ICUs. The ethical dimension is important in providing commitment and cohesion within clinical teams: pre-conditions for the development of networks.

Another factor which impinges on the development of social networks within ICUs is the lack of sophisticated models which can measure the condition of patients and provide clinicians with guidance on likely outcomes. This is not to say that there have not been attempts to devise such models. The two major models devised, to date, have focused on resources and on evaluations of severity of illness. However, whilst the output of these models may help in monitoring trends, it is not sufficiently robust to predict individual outcomes for specific cases. This is an important limitation on the use of these models: they cannot provide the basis for a sophisticated alignment of the cost of providing care with the clinical activity in the ICU. As a consequence, financial models provide crude budgetary constraints. The existence of crude budgetary constraints is an important precondition of the development of social networks within intensive care. Given the lack of refinement of the financial models, the activities of clinicians in their communications with finance and management staff assume a new significance. In exchanges with management the clinicians become the sole providers of expert advice; it must be remembered that this is advice which cannot be measured. This eliminates, on clinical grounds, crude budgetary information as a *hard* constraint.

In terms of the functioning of these networks, we depict two contrasting scenarios. Within the ICUs in the study, there is a strong commitment and a shared purpose which fits Granovetter's model of stable sub-groups in hospitals. This strength of shared purpose in these multi-disciplinary teams (the 'network') facilitates the challenging of binding constraints, and their relaxation, to permit *soft rationing* to develop. In all of these ICU teams the immediate constraint is physical, that is, the number of staffed beds. If accepted passively this would constitute a *hard rationing* situation for these ICUs. The ICU teams, however, work hard at maximising their bed usage within that constraint and when the ICU is full to capacity, they cascade patients into High Dependency Units or to recovery areas. If they still face a binding physical constraint, they can transfer patients to one of the other hospitals in this study. All these hospitals are in close proximity. In terms of financial constraints, the clinicians engage with finance staff and in effect, the finance staff become virtual members of the network. This has resulted in the financial deficit in these ICUs becoming consolidated with their budgets.

These social networks, however, work at two levels. There are tight, socially cohesive, highly democratic multi-disciplinary teams working within ICUs. But there is also a weaker social network, based on the clinicians in the ICUs in different hospitals. This is not such a tightly functioning group which meets regularly. At this level, however, the network exhibits the characteristics of weak connections in terms of contacts, but demonstrates the Granovetter thesis, that weak ties can often lead to strong network actions. We saw strong network action where these three ICUs combined successfully to engage with management in order to gain additional resources to relax the physical constraint of the number of ICU bed spaces available within the region.

Rationing is often thought of as a constraint which does or does not exist. In this chapter we have presented a more complex analysis. The acceptance of rationing fits with the notion that it is either present or not. However, the actions of the key agents within the clinical activity of intensive care may lift the constraints which apparently bind clinicians, and thus *hard rationing* becomes *soft rationing*. The success of clinical networks is now recognised by NHS management (NHS Management Executive 1999) as they seek to formalise the role of clinical networks in the management of health care. However, the direct translation of the complex social structure of networks into a management tool may prove to be problematic, because the formal adoption of the idea of networks does not recognise the strength of weak ties.

Acknowledgement

The authors acknowledge the financial support of the Research Foundation of the Chartered Institute of Management Accountants.

Notes

1 Outturn refers to actual financial results, as opposed to predicted or planned financial results
2 These are bodies, normally statutory, which are responsible for audit and accountability arrangements

References

Accounts Commission (1999) *Measuring Up to the Best: A Manager's Guide to Benchmarking*, Edinburgh: Accounts Commission.
Alter, C. (1990) An exploratory study of conflict and co-ordination of Inter-organisational Service Delivery Systems, *Academy of Management Journal*, 33, 3, 478–502.
Antos, J. (1992) Activity-based management for service, not for profit and governmental organisations, *Journal of Cost Management*, Summer, 13–23.
Atkinson, S., Bihari, D., Smithies, M., Daly, K., Mason, K.R. and McColl, I. (1994) Identification of futility in intensive care, *The Lancet*, 344, 1203–6.
Birnbaum, M.L. (1986) Cost-containment in critical care, *Critical Care Medicine*, 14, 12, 1068–77.
Blumer, H. (1969) *Symbolic Interactionism*. Englewood Cliffs, NJ: Prentice Hall.
Chambliss, D. (1996) *Beyond Caring. Hospitals, Nurses and the Social Organisation of Ethics*. Chicago University Press: Chicago.
Cox, A. and Thompson, I. (1998) On the appropriateness of benchmarking, *Journal of General Management*, 23, 3, 1–19.
Cullen, D., Keene, R. and Waternoux, C. (1974) Therapeutic intervention scoring system: a method for quantitative comparison of patient care, *Critical Care Medicine*, 2, 57–62.
Denzin, N.K. (1989) *Interpretive Interactionism*. Newbury Park, California: Sage.
Edbrooke, D., Hibbert, C. and Corcoran, M. (1999) *Review for NHS Executive of Adult Critical Care Services: An International Perspective*. Sheffield: MERCS, August.
Ferlie, E. and Pettigrew, A. (1996) Managing through networks: some issues and implications for the NHS, *British Journal of Management*, 781–99.
Glaser, B.G. and Strauss, A.L. (1967) *The Discovery of Grounded Theory – Strategies for Qualitative Research*. Chicago: Aldine.
Granovetter, M.S. (1973) The strength of weak ties, *American Journal of Sociology*, 78, 6, 1360–80.
Granovetter, M. (1982) The strength of weak ties: a network theory revisited. In Marsden, P. and Lin, N. (eds) *Social Structure and Network Analysis*. London: Sage.

Granovetter, M. (1985) Economic action and social structures: the problem of embeddedness, *American Journal of Sociology*, 9, 3, 481–510.

Granovetter, M. (1992) Economic institutions as social constructions: a framework for analysis, *Acta Sociologica*, 35, 3–11.

Hakansson, H. and Johanson, J. (1993) The network as a governance structure: interfirm cooperation beyond markets and hierarchies. In Grabner, E. (ed) *The Embedded Firm: on the Socioeconomics of Industrial Networks*. London: Routledge.

Hughes, E. (1971) *The Sociological Eye*. Chicago: Aldine.

Jacobs, S. (1996) Outcome scoring in intensive care. In Pace, N. and McLean, S. (eds) *Ethics and the Law in Intensive Care*. Oxford: Oxford University Press.

Johanson, J. and Mattson, L. (1991) Interorganizational relations in industrial systems: a network approach compared with the transactions-cost approach. In Thompson, G., Francis, J., Levacic, R. and Mitchell, J. (eds) *Markets, Hierarchies and Networks: The Co-ordination of Social Life*. London: Sage.

Knaus, W.A., Wagner, J. and Zimerman, S. (1981) APACHE Acute Physiological and Chronic Health Evaluation: a physiologically based classification system, *Critical Care Medicine*, 9, 581–97.

Lapsley, I. (1994) Responsibility accounting revived? Market reforms and budgetary control in health care, *Management Accounting Research* 5, 337–52.

Lapsley, I. and Llewellyn, S. (1995) Real life constructs: the exploration of organizational processes in case studies, *Management Accounting Research*, 6, 223–35.

Melia, K.M. (2001 in press) Ethical issues and the importance of consensus for the intensive care team, *Social Science and Medicine*.

Miranda, R.D., Ryan, D.W., Schaufeli, W.B. and Fidler, V. (1998) (eds) *Organization and Management of Intensive Care: a Prospective Study in 12 European Countries*. Berlin: Springer.

NHS Management Executive (1999) *Introduction of Managed Clinical Networks within the NHS in Scotland*. The Scottish Office: Department of Health, NHS MEL (1999) 10.

Powell, W.W. (1991) Neither market nor hierarchy: network forms of organisation. In Thompson, G., Frances, J., Levacic, R. and Mitchell, J. (eds) *Markets, Hierarchies and Networks: the Co-Ordination of Social Life*. London: Sage.

Rothman, D.J. (1992) Rationing life, *The New York Review*, 5 March, 32–7.

Singer, D.E., Carr, P.L., Mulley, A.G. and Thibault, G.E. (1983) Rationing intensive care – physician responses to a resource shortage, *The New England Journal of Medicine*, 309, 1155–60.

Spivack, D. (1987) The high cost of acute health care: a review of escalating costs and limitations of such exposure in intensive care units, *American Review of Respiratory Diseases*, 136, 1007–11.

Swenson, M. D. (1992) Scarcity in the intensive care unit: principles of justice for rationing ICU beds, *The American Journal of Medicine*, 3 May, 551–5.

Yin, R.K. (1994 Revised Edition) *Case Study Research, Design and Methods*. London: Sage.

Zussman, R. (1992) *Intensive Care: Medical Ethics and the Medical Profession*. Chicago: University of Chicago Press.

Index

Printed and bound by CPI Group (UK) Ltd, Croydon, CR0 4YY

27/10/2024

14580385-0002